Intercollegiate MRCS

Applied Basic Science

MCQs

PASTEST
Dedicated to your success

Intercollegiate MRCS

Applied Basic Science

MCQS

Christopher L H Chan BSc (Hons) MB BS FRCS
Consultant General and Colorectal Surgeon
Barts and The London
Queen Mary's School of Medicine and Dentistry
University of London

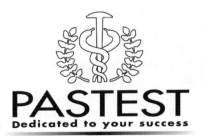

PASTEST
Dedicated to your success

© 2004 PASTEST LTD
Egerton Court
Parkgate Estate
Knutsford
Cheshire WA16 8DX

Telephone: 01565 752000

A percentage of the questions were previously published in *MRCS System Modules: The Complete Test* and *MRCS Core Modules: The Complete Test*.

First edition 2004
ISBN 1 904627 39 0

A catalogue record for this book is available from the British Library.

The information contained within this book was obtained by the author from reliable sources. However, while every effort has been made to ensure its accuracy, no responsibility for loss, damage or injury occasioned to any person acting or refraining from action as a result of information contained herein can be accepted by the publisher or author.

PasTest Revision Books and Intensive Courses

PasTest has been established in the field of postgraduate medical education since 1972, providing revision books and intensive study courses for doctors preparing for their professional examinations.
Books and courses are available for the following specialties:
MRCP Part 1 and Part 2, MRCPCH Part 1 and Part 2, MRCOG, DRCOG, MRCGP, MRCPsych, DCH, FRCA, MRCS and PLAB.
For further details contact:
**PasTest Ltd, Freepost, Knutsford, Cheshire WA16 7BR
Tel: 01565 752000   Fax: 01565 650264
E-mail: enquiries@pastest.co.uk
Web site: www.pastest.co.uk**

Typeset by Breeze Limited, Manchester
Printed by Alden Group Limited, Oxfordshire

CONTENTS

PREFACE

This book is primarily intended for candidates sitting the Part 1 (Applied Basic Sciences) section of the Intercollegiate Membership examination of the Surgical Royal Colleges of Great Britain and Ireland (MRCS). The multiple true false questions have been specifically structured to reflect the new changes in the syllabus and examination of the Surgical Royal Colleges of Great Britain and Ireland.

The goal of such a book is to help assess knowledge and provide an adjunct to reading, in addition to alerting one to areas that require further study. This book covers many of the 'most popular' topics that appear in the MRCS examination. MCQ practice will increase overall knowledge and detailed explanations have been written to aid revision. The explanations will also be useful to candidates in other parts of the examination.

I hope that this book will not be restricted only to candidates sitting the MRCS examination but will be of use to Final Year medical students.

Christopher L H Chan

CONTRIBUTORS

Editor:

Christopher L H Chan BSc (Hons) MB BS FRCS, Consultant General and Colorectal Surgeon, Barts and The London, Queen Mary's School of Medicine and Dentistry, University of London

Contributors:

Robert Attaran BSc (Hons), MBChB (Hons), University of Arizona Affiliated Hospitals, Tucson, Arizona, USA

Stuart Enoch MBBS MRCSEd MRCS (Eng), PhD Research Fellow of the Royal Colleges of Surgeons of Edinburgh and Ireland

Patrick Jassar FRCS (Ed), FRCS (ORL) Senior Fellow in Otolaryngology, Royal Darwin Hospital, Australia

Contributors to previous edition:

Steven J Arnold MSc (Hons), MRCS (Eng), East Surrey Hospital, Redhill, Surrey

Sunil Auplish MBBS, BSc (Hons), MRCS, Orthopaedic SpR, Oxford rotation

Philip J Blackie BSc (Hons), MBBS (London), Senior House Officer in Anaesthetics, King's College Hopital, London

Victoria Chamberlain MB ChB, MRCS, Wellington Hospital, Wellington, New Zealand

Joseph A Dawson MBBS MRCS (Eng), Basic Surgical Trainee, The Warwickshire & Worcestershire Basic Surgical Training Scheme

Richard J D Hewitt BSc MBBS, Senior House Officer in Neurosurgery, St Bartholomew's and the London Hospitals, London

Kismet Hossain-Ibrahim MBBS, BSc (Hons), MRCS (Eng), MRCS (Ed), Research Assistant, Department of Anatomy, University College London

Stephen J Washington MB ChB, Senior House Officer in Plastic Surgery, Christie Hospital, Manchester

EXAMINATION TECHNIQUE

The MCQ section of the new Intercollegiate Membership examination of the Surgical Royal Colleges of Great Britain and Ireland has undergone recent revision (2004) and now comprises two written papers: Part 1 for Applied Basic Sciences (ABS) and Part 2 for Clinical Problem Solving (CPS). The Part 1 ABS paper consists of multiple true false questions only. Candidates are allowed 3 hours for the paper. The Part 2 CPS consists of extended matching questions only and is presently 2½ hours in length but from April 2005 will last 3 hours.

Pacing yourself accurately during the examination to finish on time, or with time to spare, is essential. There are two common mistakes which cause good candidates to fail the MRCS written examinations. These are neglecting to read the directions and questions carefully enough and failing to fill in the computer answer card properly. You must read the instructions given to candidates at the beginning of each section of the paper to ensure that you complete the answer sheet correctly.

You must also decide on a strategy to follow with regard to marking your answer sheet. The answer sheet is read by an automatic document reader and transfers the information to a computer. It is critical that the answer sheet is filled in clearly and accurately using the pencils provided. Failure to fill in your name and your examination correctly could result in the rejection of your paper.

Some candidates mark their answers directly onto the computer sheet as they go through the question, others prefer to make a note of their answers on the question paper, and reserve time at the end to transfer their answers onto the computer sheet. If you choose the first method, there is a chance that you may decide to change your answer after a second reading. If you do change your answer on the computer sheet, you must ensure that your original is thoroughly erased. If you choose the second method, make sure that you allow enough time to transfer your answers methodically onto the computer sheet, as rushing at this stage could introduce some costly mistakes. You will find it less confusing if you transfer your marks after you have completed each section of the examination. You must ensure that you have left sufficient time to transfer your marks from the question paper to the answer sheet. You should also be aware that no additional time will be given at the end of the examination to allow you to transfer your marks.

If you find that you have time left at the end of the examination, there can be a temptation to re-read your answers time and time again, so that even those that seemed straightforward will start to look less convincing. In this situation, first thoughts are usually best, don't alter your initial answers unless you are sure.

You must also ensure that you read the question (both stem and items) carefully. Regard each item as being independent of every other item, each referring to a specific quantum of knowledge. The item (or the stem and the item taken together) make up a statement as 'True' or 'False'. The number of stems will vary for each question. For this reason, a mark will not necessarily be required for each column of the answer sheet. For every correct answer you will gain a mark (+1). Marks will not be deducted for a wrong answer. Equally, you will not gain a mark if you mark both true and false.

For this reason you should answer every question as you have nothing to lose. If you do not know the answer to a question, you should make an educated guess – you may well get the answer right and gain a mark.

If you feel that you need to spend more time puzzling over a question, leave it and, if you have time, return to it. Make sure you have collected all the marks you can before you come back to any difficult questions.

Multiple choice questions are not designed to trick you or confuse you, they are designed to test your knowledge of medicine. Accept each question at face value.

The aim of this book is to give you practice and therefore aid revision for the Part 1 ABS paper. The broad range of questions is to test your knowledge on specific subjects.

Working through the questions in this book will help you to identify your weak subject areas. In the last few weeks before the exam it will be important for you to avoid minor unimportant areas and concentrate on the most important subject areas covered in the exam.

ABBREVIATIONS

ACE	angiotensin-converting enzyme
ACTH	adrenocorticotropic hormone
ADH	antidiuretic hormone
ADP	adenosine diphosphate
ANOVA	analysis of variance
APTT	activated partial thromboplastin time
ARDS	adult respiratory distress syndrome
ARF	acute renal failure
ASIS	anterior superior iliac spine
ATP	adenosine triphosphate
AV	atrioventricular
BXO	balanitis xerotica obliterans
C1 etc. segment	cervical spinal segment
CBD	common bile duct
CCK	cholecystokinin
CEA	carcinoembryonic antigen
CN	cranial nerve
CN Vc	anterior division of mandibular nerve
CN VII	chorda tympani
CN X	recurrent laryngeal branch
CO	cardiac output
CPP	cerebral perfusion pressure
CSF	cerebrospinal fluid
CT	computed tomography
CVP	central venous pressure
CXR	chest X-ray
1,25-DHCC	1,25-dihydroxycholecalciferol
DIC	disseminated intravascular coagulation
DVT	deep vein thrombosis
EACA	epsilon-aminocaproic acid
ECM	extracellular matrix
EDRF	endothelium-derived relaxing factor
FDP	fibrin degradation products
FEV	forced expiratory volume
FFP	fresh-frozen plasma
F_{IO_2}	concentration of inspired oxygen
FRC	functional residual capacity
FSH	follicle stimulating hormone
FVC	forced vital capacity
GFR	glomerular filtration rate

GTN	glyceryl trinitrate
GVHD	graft-versus-host disease
HCO_3^-	bicarbonate
HIV	human immunodeficiency virus
HTLV	human T-cell leukaemia viruses
ICP	intracranial pressure
IL-1	interleukin-1
INR	international normalised ratio
IPPV	intermittent positive-pressure ventilation
IVC	inferior vena cava
JVP	jugular venous pressure
kg	kilogram
L1 etc. segment	lumbar spinal segment
LH	luteinizing hormone
LMWH	low-molecular-weight heparin
M	mitosis
MI	myocardial infarction
mmol	millimoles
Nd-YAG	neodymium-yttrium aluminium garnet
NO	nitric oxide
NSAIDs	non-steroidal anti-inflammatory drugs
PAH	para-aminohippuric acid
PAOP	pulmonary artery occlusion pressure
Pap smears	Papanicolaou-stained smears
PCO_2	partial pressure of carbon dioxide
PCR	polymerase chain reaction
PEA	pulseless electrical activity
PEEP	positive end-expiratory pressure
PO_2	partial pressure of oxygen
PSA	prostate-specific antigen
PT	prothrombin time
PTH	parathyroid hormone
RB1	retinoblastoma gene
RBC	red blood cell
S1 etc. segment	sacral spinal segment
SA	sinoatrial
SD	standard deviation
SIADH	syndrome of inappropriate antidiuretic homone
SMA	superior mesenteric artery
SVC	superior vena cava
SVR	systemic vascular resistance

Abbreviations

T1 etc. segment	thoracic spinal segment
T3	tri-iodothyronine
T4	thyroxine
TF	tissue factor
TIBC	total iron binding capacity
tPA	tissue plasminogen activator
TPN	total parenteral nutrition
TSH	thyroid-stimulating hormone
TT	thrombin time
TURP	transurethral resection of prostate
UC	ulcerative colitis
vWF	von Willebrand factor

QUESTIONS

SECTION 1: ANATOMY – QUESTIONS

1.1 **The following anatomical differences in children make management of their airway more difficult than in adults**

- ❏ A   a more caudally placed larynx
- ❏ B   smaller angle of the jaw
- ❏ C   a more U-shaped epiglottis
- ❏ D   relatively larger tongue
- ❏ E   larger head size compared with the body size

1.2 **The cauda equina**

- ❏ A   begins at the lower border of L1
- ❏ B   contains mainly motor fibres
- ❏ C   begins at the subcostal plane
- ❏ D   causes pain in the legs as a common feature of injury
- ❏ E   shows a positive Babinski sign with typical injury

1.3 **Nerve injuries**

- ❏ A   damage to the spinal accessory nerve causes winging of the scapula
- ❏ B   the axillary nerve contains fibres from C6 and C7
- ❏ C   radial nerve injuries cause wrist drop
- ❏ D   a positive Froment's test is associated with median nerve injury
- ❏ E   sciatic nerve injuries are associated with a high-stepping gait

1.4 **A cervical cord injury should be suspected in an unconscious patient if there is**

- ❏ A   grimacing to pain above the clavicle
- ❏ B   increased upper body tone
- ❏ C   priapism
- ❏ D   hypotension with bradycardia
- ❏ E   ability to extend the elbow

1.5 Cerebrospinal fluid

❏ A normally has a lower protein content than plasma
❏ B flows between the third and fourth ventricles via the aqueduct of Sylvius
❏ C is sterile
❏ D is produced at a rate of 2 ml/h
❏ E is produced by the arachnoid granulations

1.6 Cerebral blood flow

❏ A fluctuates widely between a lying and a standing position
❏ B is related to intracranial pressure
❏ C is directly autoregulated to arterial P_{CO_2}
❏ D is directly autoregulated to arterial P_{O_2}
❏ E is increased in the normal subject by the administration of mannitol

1.7 Intervertebral disc collapse between L5 and S1

❏ A would crush the L5 spinal nerve
❏ B would impinge into the sacral segments of the cord
❏ C usually causes pain to radiate over the medial malleolus
❏ D would exaggerate the tendon reflex at the ankle
❏ E may cause reduced sweating over the posterior aspect of the calf

1.8 A femoral nerve injury would result in

❏ A absence of the knee jerk reflex
❏ B anaesthesia over the skin of the anterior aspect of the lower leg
❏ C absence of the cremasteric reflex
❏ D paraesthesia of the skin over the medial malleolus
❏ E paraesthesia over the entire L2 dermatome

1.9 The odontoid peg

❏ A is connected to C1 by a transverse ligament
❏ B is connected to the occiput by the alar ligament
❏ C is seen on 'open mouth' view X-ray
❏ D fracture causes a retropharyngeal haematoma
❏ E has notochord remnant superiorly

1.10   Injury to the radial nerve in the radial (spiral) groove of the humerus causes loss of

❏   A   abduction of the thumb
❏   B   extension of the forearm
❏   C   supination
❏   D   cutaneous sensation over the dorsal surface of the first web space
❏   E   the brachioradialis tendon reflex

1.11   The posterior cord of the brachial plexus

❏   A   gives off the suprascapular nerve
❏   B   gives off branches to the shoulder joint
❏   C   supplies the deltoid muscle
❏   D   continues on as the radial nerve
❏   E   gives a supply to the coracobrachialis muscle

1.12   Signs of S1 nerve root compression include

❏   A   claw toes
❏   B   weakness of the extensor hallucis longus
❏   C   weakness of plantar flexion of the ankle
❏   D   weakness of ankle dorsiflexion
❏   E   enhanced ankle jerk reflex

1.13   After damage to the ulnar nerve at the elbow there is

❏   A   anaesthesia over the skin of the thenar eminence
❏   B   loss of abduction of the index finger
❏   C   loss of adduction of the wrist
❏   D   loss of flexion of the little finger
❏   E   claw hand

1.14   Traction injury of the upper trunk of the brachial plexus results in

❏   A   loss of medial rotation of the arm
❏   B   paralysis of the deltoid muscle
❏   C   loss of cutaneous sensation over the lateral surface of the arm
❏   D   loss of supination
❏   E   extension of the forearm

1.15   The left coronary artery supplies

❏ A the majority of the left ventricle
❏ B the majority of the left atrium
❏ C the sinoatrial (SA) node in most cases
❏ D the atrioventricular (AV) node in most cases
❏ E part of the right ventricle

1.16   Concerning the first rib, the

❏ A scalenus medius is attached to the scalene tubercle
❏ B subclavian artery passes posterior to the 1st thoracic nerve root
❏ C subclavian vein passes across the 1st costochondral joint
❏ D sympathetic trunk lies anterior to the neck
❏ E subclavian vein and artery are separated by the scalenus anterior

1.17   The diaphragm

❏ A is able to descend after section of the phrenic nerve
❏ B is attached to the lower six costal cartilages
❏ C receives a sensory supply through the phrenic nerve
❏ D has the oesophagus piercing the right crus
❏ E has crura pierced by splanchnic nerves

1.18   When inserting an intercostal drain in the 5th intercostal space, the following structures are encountered

❏ A pectoralis major
❏ B serratus anterior
❏ C visceral pleura
❏ D parietal pleura
❏ E internal intercostal muscle
❏ F transversus abdominis

1.19   Paralysis of the left hemidiaphragm

❏ A may be caused by section of the cord below C6
❏ B may be caused by section of the left phrenic nerve alone
❏ C causes flattening of the diaphragm during inspiration
❏ D causes paradoxical movement
❏ E increases intrathoracic pressure on the left
❏ F may occur with carcinoma of the bronchus

1.20   Inspiration involves

❏   A   descent of the hemidiaphragms
❏   B   reduction of the vertical dimension of the chest
❏   C   upward/forward movement of the first rib
❏   D   contraction of the intercostal muscles
❏   E   the long thoracic nerve of Bell (supplying the serratus anterior)

1.21   A CT scan section through the manubriosternal joint will demonstrate

❏   A   the bifurcation of the brachiocephalic artery
❏   B   the commencement of the aortic arch
❏   C   T4 vertebral body
❏   D   the bifurcation of the trachea
❏   E   the thoracic duct crossing the midline

1.22   Bleeding from the middle meningeal artery following head injury

❏   A   mainly affects the posterior branch
❏   B   results in an extradural haematoma
❏   C   may produce ipsilateral pupillary constriction
❏   D   is usually caused by a trivial incident
❏   E   typically causes a biconvex-shaped lesion on CT

1.23   The left lung has

❏   A   ten bronchopulmonary segments
❏   B   three lobes
❏   C   three bronchial openings
❏   D   two pulmonary veins
❏   E   an arterial supply from the aorta

1.24   In the base of the skull the

❏   A   foramen magnum transmits the basilar artery
❏   B   foramen spinosum transmits the VIIth cranial nerve (CN VII)
❏   C   foramen rotundum transmits the maxillary nerve
❏   D   foramen ovale transmits the greater petrosal nerve
❏   E   foramen lacerum transmits the mandibular nerve

1.25   In the main bronchial airways

❑ A   the left bronchus is longer than the right
❑ B   the right main bronchus has a wider diameter than the left
❑ C   aspiration pneumonitis is more common in the right lower lobe than the left
❑ D   the left main bronchus divides before entering the lung
❑ E   foreign bodies lodge more commonly in the right than in the left main bronchus

1.26   The recurrent laryngeal nerve

❑ A   supplies the cricothyroid muscle
❑ B   partially supplies the trachea
❑ C   lies alongside the inferior thyroid artery
❑ D   should be retracted during tracheostomy to avoid damage
❑ E   runs between the oesophagus and trachea in the neck
❑ F   supplies the mucous surface of the vocal cords

1.27   The external jugular vein

❑ A   receives a branch from the retromandibular vein
❑ B   lies anterior to scalenus anterior
❑ C   joins the subclavian vein
❑ D   has no valves
❑ E   pierces the deep cervical fascia

1.28   When the left main bronchus is dissected, the following structures may be encountered

❑ A   phrenic nerve
❑ B   vagus nerve
❑ C   recurrent laryngeal nerve
❑ D   azygos vein
❑ E   aorta

1.29   The right coronary artery

❑ A   originates in the anterior aortic sinus
❑ B   is overlain by the right atrial appendage
❑ C   supplies the sinoatrial node
❑ D   lies on the infundibulum of the right ventricle
❑ E   anastomoses with branches of the left coronary artery

1.30 The right atrium

- ❏ A forms the right border of the heart
- ❏ B lies in front of the left atrium
- ❏ C has the coronary sinus opening above the septal cusp of the tricuspid valve
- ❏ D has a posterior wall formed by the interatrial septum
- ❏ E has the sinoatrial node medial to the sulcus terminalis

1.31 The diaphragm

- ❏ A has a left crus attached to the L3 vertebra
- ❏ B is pierced by the splanchnic nerves
- ❏ C has an arterial supply from the abdominal aorta
- ❏ D has a lateral arcuate ligament overlain by the kidney
- ❏ E is related to the suprarenal glands

1.32 When the right main bronchus is dissected, the following structures may be encountered

- ❏ A the right phrenic nerve
- ❏ B the right vagus nerve
- ❏ C the right recurrent laryngeal nerve
- ❏ D the hemiazygos nerve
- ❏ E the azygos vein

1.33 Branches of the subclavian arteries supply the

- ❏ A thyroid gland
- ❏ B breast
- ❏ C rectus abdominis muscle
- ❏ D brainstem
- ❏ E diaphragm

1.34 The hilum of the left lung

- ❏ A has the phrenic nerve lying anterior to it
- ❏ B has the vagus nerve lying posterior to it
- ❏ C contains upper and lower lobe bronchi
- ❏ D is separated from the aortic arch by the vagus nerve
- ❏ E has the pulmonary artery anterior to the main bronchus

1.35   **The central tendon of the diaphragm is pierced by the**

❏   A   oesophagus
❏   B   vagus nerve
❏   C   inferior vena cava
❏   D   greater splanchnic nerves
❏   E   right phrenic nerve
❏   F   aorta
❏   G   azygos vein

1.36   **The aortic arch**

❏   A   lies anterior to the brachiocephalic veins
❏   B   gives attachment to the pretracheal fascia
❏   C   arches directly over the right pulmonary artery
❏   D   arches above the manubriosternal joint
❏   E   is covered by pleura

1.37   **The left phrenic nerve**

❏   A   carries sympathetic fibres to the diaphragm
❏   B   lies on the fibrous pericardium
❏   C   innervates the peritoneum
❏   D   originates from the C5 segment of the spinal cord
❏   E   enters the chest anterior to the subclavian vein

1.38   **The surface of the right lung is indented by the**

❏   A   trachea
❏   B   oesophagus
❏   C   superior vena cava
❏   D   right ventricle
❏   E   subclavian vein

1.39   **The trachea**

❏   A   is palpable
❏   B   bifurcates behind the manubriosternal joint
❏   C   has a left main bronchus more vertical than the right
❏   D   has a left main bronchus that branches outside the hilum
❏   E   is innervated by the recurrent laryngeal nerve

1.40   The mammary gland

❏ A   is mainly supplied by the lateral thoracic artery
❏ B   predominantly drains to the internal thoracic nodes
❏ C   partly lies on the external oblique muscle
❏ D   contains five main lactiferous ducts that drain separately at the nipple
❏ E   is a modified sebaceous gland

1.41   The breast

❏ A   has an arterial supply derived from the axillary artery
❏ B   is drained by the internal thoracic vein
❏ C   has a nipple in the T3 dermatome
❏ D   drains 60% of its lymph via the axillary lymph nodes
❏ E   has a retromammary space over the pectoralis minor muscle

1.42   In axillary lymph node dissection

❏ A   the medial wall of the axilla is formed by serratus anterior
❏ B   the clavipectoral fascia on the edge of pectoralis major should be divided to enter the axilla
❏ C   inadvertent division of the thoracodorsal nerve may lead to a winged scapula
❏ D   level II nodes are those lying lateral to pectoralis minor
❏ E   an anaesthetic patch on the medial aspect of the upper arm is a recognised complication

1.43   The lymphatic drainage of the female breast

❏ A   crosses the midline
❏ B   crosses the diaphragm
❏ C   drains to interpectoral nodes
❏ D   drains into the subclavian vein
❏ E   drains to external mammary nodes

1.44   The thoracic duct

❏ A   lies on the posterior intercostal vessels
❏ B   has no valves
❏ C   runs through the thoracic inlet to the left of the oesophagus
❏ D   receives the right bronchomediastinal lymph trunk
❏ E   arches over the left suprapleural membrane

1.45   The right phrenic nerve

❏   A   originates from nerve roots C3, C4 and C5
❏   B   is purely motor
❏   C   lies anterior to the scalenus anterior muscle
❏   D   gives off the right recurrent laryngeal nerve at the level of the right subclavian artery
❏   E   lies lateral to the right vagus nerve in the thorax

1.46   After damage to the common peroneal nerve there is

❏   A   failure of the foot to clear the ground on walking
❏   B   loss of cutaneous sensation over the sole of the foot
❏   C   weakness of inversion of the foot
❏   D   wasting of muscles in the anterior compartment of the calf
❏   E   collapse of the transverse arch of the foot

1.47   The sympathetic chain

❏   A   lies on the heads of the ribs
❏   B   lies anterior to the posterior intercostal vessels
❏   C   lies medial to the splanchnic nerves
❏   D   receives white rami communicantes from all the thoracic nerve roots
❏   E   passes into the abdomen behind the lateral arcuate ligament

1.48   The first rib

❏   A   has the scalenus anterior muscle inserting into its tubercule
❏   B   has the subclavian vein overlying the vertebral transverse processes
❏   C   has the subclavian vein running behind scalenus anterior
❏   D   is related to the pleura
❏   E   is related to the cervicothoracic ganglion
❏   F   is related to the upper two roots of the brachial plexus

1.49   The oesophagus

❏   A   is formed at the lower border of the cricoid cartilage
❏   B   passes through the central tendon of the diaphragm
❏   C   receives a sensory nerve supply from the phrenic nerve
❏   D   lies behind the right atrium
❏   E   is crossed anteriorly by the right main bronchus

1.50   The clavipectoral fascia is

❏   A   pierced by the basilic vein
❏   B   split to enclose the pectoralis major muscle
❏   C   pierced by the medial pectoral nerves
❏   D   overlain by the infraclavicular lymph nodes
❏   E   overlain by the C4 dermatome

1.51   The left brachiocephalic vein drains the

❏   A   cervical vertebrae
❏   B   bronchi
❏   C   intercostal spaces
❏   D   thoracic duct
❏   E   thyroid gland

1.52   Boundaries of the femoral triangle include

❏   A   the inguinal ligament
❏   B   adductor longus
❏   C   adductor magnus
❏   D   pectineus
❏   E   iliopsoas

1.53   The greater sciatic foramen contains the

❏   A   superior gluteal nerve
❏   B   sacrotuberous ligament
❏   C   pudendal nerve
❏   D   obturator internus tendon
❏   E   posterior femoral cutaneous nerve

1.54   In the femoral region the

❏   A   femoral sheath contains the femoral vessels
❏   B   femoral canal lies lateral to the femoral vein
❏   C   femoral canal contains Cloquet's lymph node
❏   D   femoral ring is the abdominal end of the femoral canal
❏   E   pubic branch of the inferior epigastric vein replaces the obturator vein in 30% of cases

1.55   A positive left Trendelenburg test may be associated with

❏   A   an injury to the right gluteus medius muscle
❏   B   a displaced left femoral head
❏   C   a shortened right femur
❏   D   an injury to the left abductor muscles
❏   E   an injury to the left pectineus muscle

1.56   In the popliteal fossa the

❏   A   roof is formed by the fascia lata
❏   B   sciatic nerve divides into tibial and common peroneal branches at the apex
❏   C   deepest structure is the popliteal vein
❏   D   common peroneal nerve is overlain by the semitendinosus muscle
❏   E   roof is pierced by the saphenous nerve

1.57   In the bony pelvis the

❏   A   sacral cornua are palpable per rectum
❏   B   pubic tubercles are palpable lateral to the external ring of the inguinal canal
❏   C   femoral canals lie medial to the lacunar ligaments
❏   D   ischial spines are palpable per vaginam
❏   E   transtubercular plane passes through the spinous process of the L3 vertebra

1.58   The scaphoid bone

❏   A   articulates with the radius
❏   B   is palpable in the 'snuffbox'
❏   C   has a vascular supply penetrating its distal surface
❏   D   gives attachment to the flexor retinaculum
❏   E   gives attachment to the adductor pollicis muscle

1.59   **On the dorsum of the foot the**

❑   A   dorsalis pedis artery lies medial to the extensor hallucis longus tendon
❑   B   deep peroneal nerve lies medial to the dorsalis pedis artery
❑   C   L5 dermatome is present
❑   D   great saphenous vein lies anterior to the medial malleolus
❑   E   inferior extensor retinaculum loops under the medial longitudinal arch

1.60   **In the lumbosacral plexus the**

❑   A   sympathetic trunk sends grey rami to all roots
❑   B   parasympathetic nerves originate from S2/3 spinal segments
❑   C   lumbosacral trunk lies on the piriformis muscle
❑   D   lumbosacral trunk underlies the common iliac vessels
❑   E   posterior divisions of anterior rami supply the adductor muscles

1.61   **The serratus anterior muscle**

❑   A   has the thoracodorsal nerve deep to its fascia over its lateral surface
❑   B   rotates the scapula
❑   C   retracts the scapula
❑   D   receives its nerve supply from the upper trunk of the brachial plexus
❑   E   has most of its fibres inserted into the superior angle of the scapula

1.62   **The L3 vertebra**

❑   A   undergoes rotatory movements
❑   B   gives attachment to the left crus of the diaphragm
❑   C   is supplied by the internal iliac arteries
❑   D   has a vertebral foramen (central canal) enclosing the sacral segments of the spinal cord
❑   E   has a lateral process giving attachment to the iliolumbar ligament

1.63   In the antecubital fossa the

❑ A   median nerve lies lateral to the brachial artery
❑ B   brachial artery branches into radial and ulnar arteries
❑ C   posterior interosseous nerve may be found
❑ D   cephalic vein overlies the bicipital aponeurosis
❑ E   floor is formed by the brachioradialis muscle

1.64   The carpal tunnel contains the

❑ A   median nerve
❑ B   ulnar nerve
❑ C   flexor digitorum brevis tendon
❑ D   flexor carpi ulnaris tendon
❑ E   flexor carpi radialis tendon

1.65   In the femoral triangle the

❑ A   cribriform fascia transmits the superficial branches of the femoral
         artery
❑ B   femoral vein lies adjacent to the femoral nerve
❑ C   profunda femoris artery lies medial to the femoral artery
❑ D   femoral sheath extends up to 3 cm beyond the inguinal ligament
❑ E   deep inguinal nodes lie medial to the femoral vein

1.66   The patellar reflex is

❑ A   lost after femoral nerve transection
❑ B   mediated through the posterior divisions of anterior rami of
         lumbar nerves
❑ C   lost following T12 cord transection
❑ D   present after L2–L4 dorsal root avulsions
❑ E   absent after dorsal column demyelination

1.67   The biceps tendon reflex tests the integrity of the

❑ A   musculocutaneous nerve
❑ B   medial cord of the brachial plexus
❑ C   C5 spinal segment
❑ D   C6 dorsal root
❑ E   middle trunk of the brachial plexus

1.68   The fingers are extended after

❏   A   contraction of the lumbrical muscles
❏   B   contraction of the interosseous muscles
❏   C   motor stimulation through the posterior cord of the brachial plexus
❏   D   motor stimulation through palmar digital branches of the median nerve
❏   E   motor stimulation through the ulnar nerve

1.69   A deep laceration into the thenar eminence could damage the

❏   A   superficial palmar arterial arch
❏   B   muscular recurrent branch of the median nerve
❏   C   radial artery
❏   D   flexor digitorum superficialis tendons
❏   E   adductor pollicis muscle

1.70   During full abduction of the arm the following muscles are active

❏   A   infraspinatus
❏   B   trapezius
❏   C   supraspinatus
❏   D   serratus anterior
❏   E   teres major

1.71   In a patient with a prolapsed L5/S1 intervertebral disc

❏   A   there may be no history of trauma
❏   B   pain radiating to the buttocks implies nerve root involvement
❏   C   pain radiating down to the ankle on coughing and sneezing implies nerve root involvement
❏   D   urinary retention can be secondary to pain and bedrest
❏   E   an absent ankle jerk means that the disc should be removed

1.72   The following structures exit the greater sciatic foramen below the piriformis muscle

❏   A   superior gluteal nerve and artery
❏   B   nerve to obturator internus
❏   C   femoral cutaneous nerve
❏   D   inferior gluteal nerve
❏   E   posterior cutaneous nerve of the thigh

1.73   The tibial nerve in the popliteal fossa

❏   A   runs superficial to the popliteal vessels
❏   B   emerges medial to the popliteal artery
❏   C   gives off the sural nerve as a branch
❏   D   supplies muscles for dorsiflexion of the ankle
❏   E   supplies the popliteus muscle
❏   F   runs deep to the gastrocnemius muscle

1.74   The inferior vena cava (IVC)

❏   A   enters the thoracic cavity at the level of T8
❏   B   commences at the level of L5
❏   C   receives bilateral gonadal venous drainage directly
❏   D   lies anterior to the aorta
❏   E   lies to the right of the aorta
❏   F   lies posterior to the caudate lobe of the liver

1.75   The middle meningeal artery

❏   A   arises from the maxillary branch of the external carotid artery
❏   B   originates in the pterygopalatine fossa
❏   C   enters the skull through the foramen ovale
❏   D   supplies the dura mater
❏   E   rupture of this artery is associated with an extradural haematoma

1.76   Direct branches of the coeliac plexus include the

❏   A   splenic artery
❏   B   hepatic artery
❏   C   superior pancreaticoduodenal artery
❏   D   right gastric artery
❏   E   gastroduodenal artery

1.77 The right common carotid artery

- [ ] A bifurcates at the level of the upper border of the cricoid cartilage
- [ ] B is a branch of the aortic arch
- [ ] C has the cervical sympathetic chain as an anterior relation
- [ ] D lies lateral to the lateral lobe of the thyroid gland
- [ ] E is separated from the phrenic nerve by the prevertebral fascia
- [ ] F is enclosed within the carotid sheath throughout

1.78 The basilic vein

- [ ] A begins on the medial side of the dorsal venous arch
- [ ] B drains into the subclavian vein
- [ ] C is accompanied by the medial cutaneous nerve of the forearm
- [ ] D pierces the deep fascia in the arm
- [ ] E lies medial to the biceps tendon in the cubital fossa

1.79 The posterior tibial artery

- [ ] A descends on the posterior surface of the tibia distally
- [ ] B gives rise to the anterior tibial artery
- [ ] C gives rise to the peroneal artery
- [ ] D passes anterior to the fibrous arch of the soleus muscle
- [ ] E passes deep to the flexor retinaculum at the ankle

1.80 The abdominal aorta

- [ ] A enters the abdomen at the level of the T12 vertebra
- [ ] B divides at the level of the L5 vertebra
- [ ] C lies to the left of the cisterna chyli
- [ ] D gives off four single ventral gut arteries
- [ ] E lies posterior to the right renal vein
- [ ] F gives rise to pulsations that are normally palpable

1.81 The femoral artery

- [ ] A underlies the inguinal ligament medial to the deep inguinal ring
- [ ] B supplies the hamstring muscles
- [ ] C supplies the head of the femur
- [ ] D passes through the adductor longus muscle
- [ ] E is subcutaneous in the femoral triangle

1.82   The portal vein

☐ A   is formed behind the body of the pancreas
☐ B   lies anteriorly to the free edge of the lesser omentum
☐ C   drains the spleen
☐ D   forms the central vein of each liver lobule
☐ E   lies to the right of the superior mesenteric artery
☐ F   is about 10 cm in length

1.83   Application of arterial clips during total thyroidectomy could injure the following nerves

☐ A   recurrent laryngeal
☐ B   internal laryngeal
☐ C   external laryngeal
☐ D   phrenic
☐ E   transverse cervical

1.84   The brachial artery is

☐ A   palpable in the arm
☐ B   crossed anteriorly by the median nerve
☐ C   overlain by the biceps tendon
☐ D   surrounded by venae comitantes
☐ E   accompanied by the ulnar nerve

1.85   The thoracic duct

☐ A   runs to the right of the descending aorta
☐ B   opens into the superior vena cava
☐ C   is anterior to the subclavian artery
☐ D   starts at the level of T10
☐ E   drains into the right subclavian vein

1.86   Lymphatic ducts

☐ A   contract due to filling
☐ B   have no valves
☐ C   if obstructed, lead to lymphoedema
☐ D   have a parasympathetic innervation
☐ E   empty by pump action of the calf muscles
☐ F   dilate in oedema

1.87   The abdominal aorta

❏   A   passes into the abdomen at the level of T12
❏   B   lies to the left of the cysterna chyli
❏   C   is anterior to the right lumbar sympathetic trunk
❏   D   gives off four paired branches
❏   E   bifurcates at the level of L5

1.88   Structures encountered on right carotid endarterectomy include the

❏   A   vagus nerve
❏   B   sympathetic chain
❏   C   cervical ganglion
❏   D   thoracic duct
❏   E   pleural membranes

1.89   The cephalic vein

❏   A   forms in the anatomical snuffbox
❏   B   is deep to the cutaneous nerve of the forearm
❏   C   joins the brachial artery at the elbow
❏   D   is medial to the biceps tendon
❏   E   forms the axillary vein by joining the basilic vein
❏   F   has no valves

1.90   The arch of the aorta

❏   A   lies wholly in the superior mediastinum
❏   B   reaches the vertebral column at the lower border of the fourth thoracic vertebra
❏   C   is crossed anteriorly by the left phrenic nerve
❏   D   gives rise to the right internal mammary artery
❏   E   gives rise to the left vertebral artery

1.91   The radial artery

❏   A   anastomoses with the ulnar artery
❏   B   passes over the trapezium in the wrist
❏   C   passes into the hand between the two heads of the adductor
          pollicis muscle
❏   D   lies lateral to the biceps tendon in the cubital fossa
❏   E   is overlain by the pronator teres muscle
❏   F   is larger than the ulnar artery

**1.92   Structures related to the superficial part of the submandibular
gland include**

❏   A   platysma
❏   B   the mandibular branch of the facial nerve
❏   C   the facial artery
❏   D   the facial vein
❏   E   deep cervical fascia

1.93   The posterior tongue contains

❏   A   vallate papillae
❏   B   lymphoid tissue
❏   C   filiform papillae
❏   D   fungiform papillae

1.94   Surgical anatomy of the thyroid

❏   A   the superior thyroid artery enters the upper pole of the thyroid
          gland close to the recurrent laryngeal nerve
❏   B   damage to the external laryngeal nerve causes loss of high-
          pitched phonation
❏   C   the inferior thyroid artery arises from the origin of the external
          carotid artery
❏   D   the inferior thyroid artery should be ligated as far laterally as
          possible
❏   E   the isthmus lies anterior to the trachea

1.95 The thyroid gland

❑ A initially moves down on swallowing
❑ B lies superficial to the myofascial layer in the neck
❑ C receives 5% of the total cardiac output
❑ D derives its arterial supply solely from branches of the external carotid
❑ E has a venous plexus draining into the internal jugular and brachiocephalic veins

1.96 The tongue

❑ A receives sensory innervation from the vagus nerve
❑ B protrudes to the side of a unilateral lower motor neurone lesion
❑ C is active during the voluntary phase of swallowing
❑ D is retracted by the hyoglossus muscle
❑ E contains lymphoid tissue
❑ F has intrinsic muscles that are not attached to any bone

1.97 The parotid gland

❑ A is encapsulated by the investing layer of deep cervical fascia
❑ B receives its blood supply directly from the external carotid artery
❑ C is traversed by the facial artery
❑ D is separated from the carotid sheath by the styloid process
❑ E contains the common facial vein
❑ F has a duct that passes anteriorly, superficial to the masseter

1.98 The submandibular gland

❑ A lies below the digastric muscle
❑ B has the hypoglossal nerve running through it
❑ C lies both below and above the lower mandible
❑ D is superficial to the hyoglossus muscle
❑ E has the facial artery running through it

1.99   The true vocal folds are

❑   A   lined by respiratory epithelium
❑   B   formed by the lower free edge of the quadrangular membranes
❑   C   abducted by the lateral cricoarytenoid muscles
❑   D   abducted by the posterior cricoarytenoid muscles
❑   E   tensed by contractions of the cricothyroid muscles
❑   F   innervated by sensory fibres of the internal laryngeal nerves

1.100   The posterior triangle of the neck contains the

❑   A   great auricular nerve
❑   B   omohyoid muscle
❑   C   supraclavicular nerves
❑   D   roots of the brachial plexus
❑   E   vertebral artery

1.101   The chorda tympani

❑   A   contains taste fibres
❑   B   is secretomotor to the parotid salivary gland
❑   C   exits the middle ear via the stylomastoid foramen
❑   D   is vulnerable to damage during parotid surgery
❑   E   is damaged by compression at the stylomastoid foramen
❑   F   joins the lingual nerve

1.102   The pituitary fossa

❑   A   can be seen on a lateral skull X-ray
❑   B   lies above the sphenoid bone
❑   C   is associated with the cavernous sinus
❑   D   lies in the middle cerebral fossa
❑   E   tumours usually press upon the posterior part of the optic
          chiasma

1.103   The recurrent laryngeal nerve

❑   A   supplies all intrinsic laryngeal muscles
❑   B   supplies the cricothyroid muscle
❑   C   supplies sensation to the subglottic region
❑   D   is sensory to the supraglottic region
❑   E   supplies the sternothyroid muscle

1.104   The middle meatus

❑   A   drains the nasolacrimal duct
❑   B   contains the bulla ethmoidalis
❑   C   drains the sphenoidal air sinus
❑   D   drains the posterior ethmoidal air sinus
❑   E   is lined by olfactory epithelium

1.105   Occlusion of the posterior cerebral artery causes

❑   A   nystagmus
❑   B   visual disturbances
❑   C   dysphasia
❑   D   contralateral hemiplegia
❑   E   bilateral homonymous hemianopia

1.06   Anatomy of the orbit

❑   A   the supraorbital nerve passes through the superior orbital fissure
❑   B   the ophthalmic artery passes through the superior orbital fissure
❑   C   the optic nerve is surrounded by pia, arachnoid and dura mater
❑   D   the frontal nerve passes through the tendinous membrane
❑   E   the nasociliary nerve supplies the cornea
❑   F   sectioning of the inferior ramus of the oculomotor nerve will produce a ptosis
❑   G   the ophthalmic artery is a branch of the internal carotid artery

1.107   Pain in the ear during acute tonsillitis is due to the

❑   A   superior laryngeal nerve
❑   B   glossopharyngeal nerve
❑   C   facial nerve
❑   D   hypoglossal nerve
❑   E   lesser palatine nerve

1.108   Infarction of the left occipital lobe would produce

❑   A   left homonymous hemianopia
❑   B   right visual field loss
❑   C   macular sparing
❑   D   blindness in the right eye
❑   E   paralysis of the lateral rectus muscle

1.109 Complications of submandibular gland excision include

❑ A weakness of the angle of the mouth
❑ B anaesthesia of the contralateral half of the tongue
❑ C deviation of the tongue to the contralateral side
❑ D Frey's syndrome
❑ E damage to the retromandibular vein

1.110 Transection of the anterior division of the mandibular nerve (CN Vc) in the infratemporal fossa results in

❑ A ipsilateral paralysis of the buccinator muscle
❑ B dysphagia
❑ C ipsilateral anaesthesia of the mandibular teeth
❑ D deviation of the jaw to the side of the lesion on protrusion
❑ E ipsilateral anaesthesia of the mucosa of the oral vestibule

1.111 On turning the head to the left

❑ A the left sternocleidomastoid muscle is the main agonist
❑ B movement takes place at the atlanto-occipital joint
❑ C neural impulses pass via the spinal accessory nerve
❑ D the axis of rotation runs vertically through the odontoid process
❑ E movement is limited by cervical vertebrae

1.112 Within the orbit

❑ A the optic nerve is invested by meninges
❑ B ischaemic necrosis of the retina follows optic nerve transection
❑ C blow-out fractures can cause diplopia
❑ D trochlear nerve lesions cause ptosis
❑ E frontal nerve lesions depress the corneal reflex

1.113 Structures superficial to the sternocleidomastoid muscle include the

❑ A transverse cervical nerve
❑ B transverse cervical artery
❑ C great auricular nerve
❑ D external jugular vein
❑ E inferior thyroid artery

1.114   The inferior thyroid artery

❑   A   supplies the inferior and superior parathyroid glands
❑   B   supplies the oesophagus
❑   C   arises from the external carotid artery
❑   D   is ligated close to the gland in a thyroidectomy
❑   E   supplies the inferior pole of the thyroid

1.115   Structures passing through the foramen magnum include

❑   A   medulla oblongata
❑   B   vertebral arteries
❑   C   spinal arteries
❑   D   vertebral veins
❑   E   dura mater

1.116   The internal jugular veins

❑   A   emerge from the posterior compartment of the jugular foramen
❑   B   drain the cavernous venous sinus
❑   C   have the ansa cervicalis as an anterior relation
❑   D   are the most anterior structures in the carotid sheath
❑   E   drain into the brachiocephalic veins behind the sternoclavicular joints
❑   F   lie deep to the sternocleidomastoid muscle

1.117   The superior vena cava (SVC)

❑   A   has a valve at its entry into the left atrium
❑   B   drains only the head, neck and upper body
❑   C   receives the thoracic duct
❑   D   ends behind the second costal cartilage
❑   E   enters the heart at the level of the sternal angle

1.118   The ophthalmic artery

❑   A   has the central artery of the retina as its terminal branch
❑   B   supplies both the anterior and posterior ethmoidal arteries
❑   C   originates from the internal carotid artery
❑   D   enters the orbit through the superior orbital fissure
❑   E   supplies the skin over the forehead
❑   F   travels with the nasociliary nerve
❑   G   supplies the cornea

1.119   The external carotid artery

❑ A   terminates at the level of the cricoid cartilage
❑ B   is crossed by the posterior belly of the digastric muscle
❑ C   lies superficial to the hypoglossal nerve
❑ D   is separated from the internal carotid artery by the
          stylopharyngeus and styloglossus muscles
❑ E   contains the carotid sinus

1.120   The spinal canal (vertebral foramen)

❑ A   is anterior to the ligamentum flavum
❑ B   is posterior to the vertebral disc
❑ C   is constant in diameter
❑ D   is lateral to the facets
❑ E   ends at L1

1.121   The thoracic duct

❑ A   lies to the right of the aorta
❑ B   opens into the superior vena cava
❑ C   is anterior to the left subclavian artery
❑ D   commences at the level of T10
❑ E   drains into the right subclavian vein

1.122   The eustachian tube in the infant

❑ A   connects the middle ear to the oropharynx
❑ B   opens by the palatine tonsil
❑ C   has a bony portion in the sphenoid bone
❑ D   has a cartilaginous medial segment
❑ E   is more horizontal than it is in the adult

1.123   Positions for an ectopic testis include

❑ A   inguinal
❑ B   penile
❑ C   intra-abdominal
❑ D   femoral
❑ E   high scrotal

1.124   Levator ani

❏   A   forms the roof of the ischiorectal fossa
❏   B   may be divided into deep and superficial parts
❏   C   is supplied by L4/L5
❏   D   origin includes the obturator fascia
❏   E   lies at the bifurcation of the aorta

1.125   The superior mesenteric artery

❏   A   supplies the whole of the jejunum and ileum
❏   B   lies to the left of the superior mesenteric vein
❏   C   lies behind the neck of the pancreas
❏   D   lies posterior to the third part of the duodenum
❏   E   lies above the splenic vein

1.126   Through the epiploic foramen the

❏   A   caudate lobe of the liver is palpable in the lesser sac
❏   B   inferior vena cava lies posteriorly
❏   C   portal vein lies anteriorly
❏   D   right gastric artery lies posteriorly
❏   E   second part of the duodenum forms the lower boundary

1.127   Borders of Hesselbach's triangle include

❏   A   the inferior epigastric artery
❏   B   the inguinal ligament
❏   C   the medial border of the rectus abdominis muscle
❏   D   the lacunar ligament
❏   E   the femoral artery

1.128   The epiploic foramen

❏   A   has the quadrate lobe of the liver as a superior boundary
❏   B   has the gastroduodenal artery lying medially
❏   C   has the portal vein lying posteriorly
❏   D   has the third part of the duodenum lying inferiorly
❏   E   is involved in Pringle's manoeuvre

1.129   The psoas muscle

❏   A   originates in part from the lumbar transverse processes
❏   B   inserts into the greater trochanter
❏   C   flexes the hip joint
❏   D   externally rotates the leg
❏   E   is supplied by the femoral nerve

1.130   The uterus

❏   A   is related to the small bowel
❏   B   has the ureters running laterally across it
❏   C   is supplied by a direct branch of the external iliac artery
❏   D   is covered completely with peritoneum
❏   E   is related to the pouch of Douglas
❏   F   is supplied by the pudendal nerves
❏   G   is supplied by the obturator nerves

1.131   The liver

❏   A   has the left lobe in direct contact with the left suprarenal gland
❏   B   is covered completely with peritoneum
❏   C   is attached to the diaphragm by the falciform ligament
❏   D   is in contact with both the oesophagus and the stomach
❏   E   has the right and left lobes divided individually into four
        vascular segments

1.132   The inferior mesenteric vein

❏   A   drains the rectum
❏   B   lies anterior to the left renal vein
❏   C   is a tributary of the portal vein
❏   D   lies to the right of the inferior mesenteric artery
❏   E   lies anterior to the left ureter
❏   F   drains the ileum

1.133   The portal vein

❑   A   is anterior to the first part of the duodenum
❑   B   is formed in the confluence of the superior mesenteric and
          splenic veins
❑   C   lies behind the epiploic foramen
❑   D   receives tributaries from the pancreatic neck
❑   E   lies partly in the lesser omentum

1.134   The inferior vena cava (IVC)

❑   A   carries most of the blood below the diaphragm back to the heart
❑   B   has the right sympathetic trunk lying behind its right margin
❑   C   receives direct tributaries from both suprarenal glands
❑   D   receives direct tributaries from both kidneys
❑   E   receives direct tributaries from both gonads
❑   F   is valveless

1.135   Portal vein thrombosis may

❑   A   occur in patients with thrombophilia
❑   B   occur after severe appendicitis
❑   C   cause small bowel infarction
❑   D   cause small intestinal varicosities
❑   E   cause splenomegaly

1.136   The internal iliac artery supplies the

❑   A   sigmoid colon
❑   B   spinal cord
❑   C   trochanteric anastomosis
❑   D   bladder
❑   E   anterior superior iliac spine anastomosis

1.137   Inguinal lymph nodes receive drainage from the

❑   A   scrotum
❑   B   testis
❑   C   cervix
❑   D   lumbosacral skin
❑   E   fallopian tubes

1.138   The superficial inguinal lymph nodes drain the

❏   A   skin of the gluteal region
❏   B   skin of the perianal region
❏   C   uterus
❏   D   testis
❏   E   skin of the dorsum of the foot

1.139   Posterior relations of the stomach include the

❏   A   right kidney
❏   B   head of the pancreas
❏   C   left psoas muscle
❏   D   left adrenal gland
❏   E   left hemidiaphragm

1.140   Relations of the intrathoracic oesophagus include the

❏   A   trachea
❏   B   left lobe of the liver
❏   C   accessory hemiazygos vein
❏   D   pericardium
❏   E   right main bronchus
❏   F   inferior vena cava

1.141   A Kocher's incision

❏   A   divides the Colles' fascia
❏   B   divides only the anterior rectus sheath
❏   C   divides the external oblique muscle
❏   D   involves the area innervated by T10 nerve root
❏   E   divides the fascia transversalis muscle
❏   F   divides the rectus abdominis muscle

1.142   The lienorenal ligament contains the

❏   A   splenic artery
❏   B   renal artery
❏   C   tail of the pancreas
❏   D   portal vein
❏   E   splenic vein
❏   F   left adrenal gland

1.143   During digital rectal examination you can feel the

- ❏ A   ischial tuberosity
- ❏ B   rectovesical pouch
- ❏ C   cervix
- ❏ D   seminal vesicles
- ❏ E   ureter

1.144   The epiploic foramen

- ❏ A   has a superior border formed by the caudate lobe of the liver
- ❏ B   has an inferior border formed by the second part of the duodenum
- ❏ C   has the aorta as a posterior border
- ❏ D   has the gastroduodenal artery as a posterior border
- ❏ E   has the portal vein lying anteriorly
- ❏ F   has the inferior vena cava lying inferiorly

1.145   In the inguinal region

- ❏ A   the pectineal ligament is also known as Astley Cooper's ligament
- ❏ B   the vas deferens is also known as the duct of Santorini
- ❏ C   the inguinal ligament is also known as Poupart's ligament
- ❏ D   the transversalis fascia is also known as Scarpa's fascia
- ❏ E   Cloquet's node lies within the femoral canal
- ❏ F   the femoral canal is also known as Alcock's canal

1.146   The right suprarenal gland

- ❏ A   lies against the bare area of the liver
- ❏ B   extends behind the inferior vena cava (IVC)
- ❏ C   receives blood from the right inferior phrenic artery
- ❏ D   drains into the right renal vein
- ❏ E   lies on the ninth rib

1.147 During inguinal hernia repair, the following structures are encountered

❑ A Scarpa's fascia
❑ B Colles' fascia
❑ C ilioinguinal nerve
❑ D cremasteric muscle
❑ E superior epigastric vein
❑ F iliohypogastric nerve

1.148 In the surgical anatomy of the liver

❑ A segment I lies to the left of the portal vein
❑ B segment II lies medial to the porta hepatis
❑ C the caudate lobe lies anterior to the portal vein
❑ D the portal vein runs in the anterior border of Winslow's foramen
❑ E three hepatic veins divide the liver into four sectors

1.149 The anal canal

❑ A lies below the levator ani muscle
❑ B has a longitudinal muscular coat
❑ C has a lymphatic drainage via the inguinal lymph nodes
❑ D has an external sphincter innervated by the pudendal nerve
❑ E possesses valves
❑ F lies behind the anococcygeal body

1.150 The mesentery of the small bowel

❑ A contains veins which drain directly into the inferior vena cava
❑ B has a root overlying the left sacroiliac joint
❑ C contains autonomic fibres of the vagus nerve
❑ D contains arteries that supply the large bowel
❑ E overlies the transverse mesocolon

1.151 The spleen

❑ A is related to the left costodiaphragmatic recess
❑ B is in contact with the pancreas
❑ C must triple in size to be palpable
❑ D is attached to the stomach by the lienorenal ligament
❑ E has the lesser sac extending into its hilum

1.152   The deep perineal pouch in men contains the

❏   A   membranous urethra
❏   B   seminal vesicles
❏   C   prostatic urethra
❏   D   sphincter urethra
❏   E   bulb of the penis
❏   F   bulbourethral glands
❏   G   middle rectal artery

1.153   In the inguinal region

❏   A   the inguinal ligament is formed by the in-rolled edge of the internal oblique aponeurosis
❏   B   the inguinal ligament runs from the anterior inferior iliac spine to the pubic symphysis
❏   C   the inguinal canal contains a nerve arising from the second and third sacral nerves.
❏   D   the inferior epigastric artery runs laterally to the deep inguinal ring
❏   E   a direct inguinal hernia arises medial to the deep inguinal ring

1.154   The external inguinal ring in a man

❏   A   is formed by a V-shaped slit in the internal oblique aponeurosis
❏   B   transmits the testicular artery
❏   C   transmits the cremasteric artery
❏   D   transmits the femoral branch of the genitofemoral nerve
❏   E   transmits the pampiniform plexus
❏   F   transmits the iliohypogastric nerve
❏   G   transmits the cremasteric muscle

1.155   The urethra in men

❏   A   has a prostatic part bounded by the internal and external urethral sphincter
❏   B   has a spongy part which, when ruptured, leaks urine over the abdomen subcutaneously
❏   C   has a 90° angle in its membranous part
❏   D   is narrowest at the external urethral meatus
❏   E   has a penile part invested by the erectile tissue of the corpora cavernosa

1.156   The prostate gland

❏   A   is traversed by ejaculatory ducts
❏   B   is lateral to levator ani
❏   C   receives a blood supply from the pudendal artery
❏   D   has the ureters lying laterally
❏   E   has a venous drainage to the internal vertebral plexus
❏   F   contains the widest part of the urethra

1.157   The posterior third of the tongue has

❏   A   filiform papillae
❏   B   fungiform papillae
❏   C   lymphoid tissue
❏   D   a sensory innervation from the internal laryngeal nerve
❏   E   a sensory innervation from the chordae tympani

1.158   The ilioinguinal nerve

❏   A   lies posterior to the kidney
❏   B   is entirely sensory
❏   C   passes through the deep inguinal ring
❏   D   passes through the superficial inguinal ring
❏   E   supplies sensation to the scrotum
❏   F   may be damaged by a grid-iron incision

1.159   The rectum

❏   A   normally drains into the superficial inguinal lymph nodes
❏   B   has a venous drainage into the superior mesenteric vein
❏   C   has a peritoneal mesentery
❏   D   drains to the mesenteric lymph nodes
❏   E   is supplied by the middle rectal artery

1.160   The kidney is in direct contact with the

❏   A   costodiaphragmatic angle of the pleural cavity
❏   B   subcostal nerve
❏   C   psoas muscle
❏   D   ilioinguinal nerve
❏   E   cisterna chyli

1.161 The femoral artery

❏ A   is anterior to the vein in the adductor canal
❏ B   has no branch in the adductor canal
❏ C   is posterior to the psoas muscle
❏ D   is posterior to the adductor brevis
❏ E   is posterior to the adductor longus
❏ F   passes through the adductor longus
❏ G   is posterior to the femoral vein in the upper thigh

1.162 The tibial nerve

❏ A   gives off the sural nerve
❏ B   lies superficial to the artery in the popliteal fossa
❏ C   lies lateral to the popliteal artery throughout its course
❏ D   if damaged, will result in loss of dorsiflexion of the foot
❏ E   supplies the knee joint

1.163 The linea semilunaris of the rectus sheath

❏ A   is crossed by the inferior epigastric vessels
❏ B   has an upper attachment overlying the gallbladder
❏ C   is one of the preferred lines of incision in abdominal surgery
❏ D   is formed by interdigitation of the internal and external oblique aponeuroses
❏ E   is crossed by the medial umbilical ligament
❏ F   can be involved in a spigelian hernia
❏ G   forms one side of Hesselbach's triangle

1.164 The scalp region

❏ A   is supplied exclusively from branches of the external carotid artery
❏ B   contains the C1 dermatome
❏ C   is tightly attached to the cranium
❏ D   contains lymph nodes
❏ E   has a motor innervation from the facial nerve

1.165   The third part of the duodenum lies

❑   A   posterior to the superior mesenteric vessels
❑   B   immediately anterior to the right renal artery
❑   C   posterior to the root of the mesentery of the small bowel
❑   D   anterior to the right ureter
❑   E   anterior to the inferior mesenteric artery

1.166   The pancreas

❑   A   overlies the right kidney
❑   B   lies in the transpyloric plane
❑   C   has an uncinate process lying anterior to the superior mesenteric vein
❑   D   gives attachment to the transverse mesocolon
❑   E   has the inferior mesenteric vein passing behind the neck

1.167   A patient presents with numbness in the first, second and third toes. The nerves contributing to the numbness include

❑   A   the medial plantar nerve
❑   B   the lateral plantar nerve
❑   C   the superficial peroneal nerve
❑   D   the sural nerve

1.168   Compared with the lower end of the ileum, the upper end of the jejunum has

❑   A   a thicker wall
❑   B   less fat at the mesenteric border
❑   C   fewer circular folds
❑   D   a wider lumen
❑   E   more aggregated lymphatic follicles (Peyer's patches)
❑   F   more arterial arcades

1.169   The spermatic cord contains the

❑   A   pampiniform plexus
❑   B   vas deferens
❑   C   testicular artery
❑   D   dartos muscles
❑   E   femoral branch of the genitofemoral nerve
❑   F   ilioinguinal nerve

1.170   The medial ligament of the ankle

❑ A   comprises three separate bands
❑ B   is damaged in a 'sprained' ankle
❑ C   inserts into the calcaneum
❑ D   has a superficial part
❑ E   may be associated with an avulsion fracture on X-ray

1.171   The abdominal inferior vena cava (IVC)

❑ A   runs in the free edge of the lesser omentum
❑ B   ascends to the right of the aorta
❑ C   may be directly in contact with the right suprarenal gland
❑ D   forms the posterior wall of the epiploic foramen
❑ E   receives direct drainage from both the right and left suprarenal veins

1.172   The processus vaginalis

❑ A   is formed by visceral peritoneum
❑ B   forms a sac in which the testis descends through the inguinal canal
❑ C   when present in adults, predisposes to direct inguinal hernia
❑ D   forms the tunica vaginalis in the adult
❑ E   invests the adult vas deferens

1.173   The adductor canal

❑ A   is bounded in part by the vastus lateralis
❑ B   contains the saphenous nerve
❑ C   contains the deep femoral artery
❑ D   contains the nerve to the vastus medialis
❑ E   contains an artery that forms an anastomosis around the knee joint
❑ F   contains the nerve that supplies tensor fascia lata

1.174   The typical rib has

❑ A   an angle at its anterior end
❑ B   a costal groove on its superior border
❑ C   a tubercle between the head and neck
❑ D   an articulation with two vertebrae
❑ E   an angle which is the likeliest part to fracture in thoracic trauma

1.175   The axillary artery

❏   A   has branches in its first part
❏   B   passes through deep fascia
❏   C   is a continuation of the subclavian artery
❏   D   and all its branches are usually encountered in an axillary dissection
❏   E   commences at the lateral border of the second rib

1.176   The lesser omentum

❏   A   is supplied by gastroepiploic arteries
❏   B   is attached to the liver in the fissure of the ligamentum venosum
❏   C   encloses the right gastric vessels
❏   D   has the common hepatic bile duct in its free edge
❏   E   is attached to the first part of the duodenum
❏   F   has considerable mobility

1.177   The following are found during an approach to the right subclavian artery

❏   A   stellate ganglion
❏   B   vagus nerve
❏   C   phrenic nerve
❏   D   scalenus anterior
❏   E   thoracic duct

1.178   In the female reproductive tract

❏   A   the ovarian artery supplies the fallopian tube
❏   B   most of the anterior surface of the uterus is covered by peritoneum
❏   C   ureteric calculi are palpable per vaginam
❏   D   the ovary lies posterior to the broad ligament
❏   E   lymph drains from the uterine tubes to the superficial inguinal lymph nodes
❏   F   the major arterial supply of the uterus originates from the internal iliac artery
❏   G   the suspensory ligament of the ovary is a remnant of the gubernaculum

1.179   The lower urinary tract

- ❏ A   receives a parasympathetic supply from S2–S4
- ❏ B   is supplied by the obturator nerve
- ❏ C   receives a sympathetic supply via the hypogastric plexus
- ❏ D   is supplied by the perineal branch of the pudendal nerve
- ❏ E   has the detrusor muscle under parasympathetic control

1.180   An abscess in the temporal lobe may cause

- ❏ A   epilepsy
- ❏ B   visual disturbances
- ❏ C   problems with balance
- ❏ D   problems with speech recognition
- ❏ E   meningitis

1.181   The cephalic vein

- ❏ A   forms in the area of the anatomical snuffbox
- ❏ B   is deep to the cutaneous nerve of the forearm
- ❏ C   is medial to the biceps muscle
- ❏ D   forms the axillary vein by joining the basilic vein
- ❏ E   lies on the ulnar aspect of the wrist
- ❏ F   has no valves

1.182   The middle ear

- ❏ A   has the facial nerve running through its roof
- ❏ B   is lined with a mucous membrane
- ❏ C   contains all the auditory ossicles
- ❏ D   has the internal carotid artery running anteriorly
- ❏ E   has a promontory in the projection of the lateral semicircular canal
- ❏ F   has the internal jugular vein running medially

1.183   The palatine tonsillar bed

- ❏ A   lies in the oral cavity
- ❏ B   is floored by the middle constrictor muscle
- ❏ C   contains the superior pharyngeal nerve
- ❏ D   is pierced by branches of the facial artery
- ❏ E   is drained by the external palatine vein

1.184 The ischiorectal fossae

❑ A communicate across the midline
❑ B contain the inferior rectal branches of the pudendal nerve
❑ C have a base formed by skin
❑ D have anterior recesses above the perineal membrane
❑ E contain the internal pudendal vessels

1.185 In the gluteal region, the sciatic nerve lies

❑ A on the piriformis muscle
❑ B deep in the upper outer quadrant
❑ C on the capsule of the hip joint
❑ D medial to the inferior gluteal vessels
❑ E anterior to the obturator internus muscle

1.186 Intimate relations of the left recurrent laryngeal nerve include the

❑ A oesophagus
❑ B trachea
❑ C left subclavian artery
❑ D ligamentum arteriosum
❑ E inferior thyroid artery

1.187 The right renal artery

❑ A branches several times before entering the kidney
❑ B gives a branch to the ureter
❑ C lies anterior to the renal vein
❑ D lies anterior to the inferior vena cava

1.188 The ureter

❑ A is supplied by lumbar arteries
❑ B lies anterior to the gonadal vessels
❑ C is crossed anteriorly by the vas deferens
❑ D lies over the external iliac artery in its distal third
❑ E has a nerve supply to its upper third from the T10 segment of the spinal cord

1.189   At the knee joint

❏   A   the popliteus tendon is intracapsular
❏   B   the suprapatellar bursa communicates with the joint
❏   C   the iliotibial tract inserts into the fibula
❏   D   the anterior cruciate ligament is supplied by the middle
            geniculate artery
❏   E   rotation occurs below the menisci

1.190   The trigeminal nerve

❏   A   supplies the buccinator muscle
❏   B   supplies the muscles of mastication
❏   C   has ophthalmic and maxillary divisions, which are only sensory
❏   D   is sensory to the temporomandibular joint
❏   E   supplies sensation to the angle of the mandible

1.191   Cervical rib

❏   A   most commonly produces arterial symptoms
❏   B   may produce a bruit in the supraclavicular fossa
❏   C   causes paraesthesiae most commonly in the C6 nerve root
            distribution
❏   D   is bilateral in 50% of cases
❏   E   is not associated with arm swelling

1.192   The base of the bladder lies on the

❏   A   seminal vesicles
❏   B   ureters
❏   C   ductus (vas) deferens
❏   D   anterior vaginal wall
❏   E   cervix

1.193   Posterior relations of the right kidney include the

❏   A   psoas muscle
❏   B   subcostal nerve
❏   C   peritoneum
❏   D   diaphragm
❏   E   right suprarenal gland

1.194   In surgical anatomy of the thyroid gland

❏   A   the thyroid gland has a definite, fine capsule
❏   B   Berry's ligament connects the thyroid to the cricoid cartilage and upper trachea
❏   C   the inferior parathyroid glands are more constant in position than the superior parathyroid glands
❏   D   the middle thyroid veins are more constant in position than the superior and inferior thyroid veins
❏   E   unilateral recurrent laryngeal nerve division results in the contralateral vocal cord lying in the mid- or cadaveric position

1.195   Transection of the cervical part of the sympathetic chain at the root of the neck results in

❏   A   vasomotor changes in the arm
❏   B   ptosis
❏   C   pupillary dilatation
❏   D   ablation of sympathetic supply to the pulmonary plexus
❏   E   loss of sweating over the C4 dermatome

1.196   The trachea

❏   A   begins at the level of the thyroid cartilage
❏   B   is in contact with the right pleura
❏   C   has fibroelastic cartilage in its wall
❏   D   is innervated by the recurrent laryngeal nerve
❏   E   is in contact with the left common carotid artery

1.197   The prostate gland

❏   A   is pierced by the ducts of the seminal vesicles
❏   B   has a venous plexus contained within its capsule
❏   C   lies below the urogenital diaphragm
❏   D   contains the membranous urethra
❏   E   is separated from the rectum by peritoneum

1.198   Relations of the pituitary include the

❑   A   diaphragma sellae
❑   B   optic chiasma
❑   C   sphenoid sinus
❑   D   temporal lobe
❑   E   cavernous sinus

1.199   At the ankle joint the

❑   A   peroneus tertius tendon grooves the lateral malleolus
❑   B   flexor digitorum longus tendon grooves the medial malleolus
❑   C   deltoid ligament is attached to the calcaneus
❑   D   posterior tibial artery lies between the tibialis posterior and
           flexor digitorum longus tendons
❑   E   tibial nerve lies anterior to the posterior tibial artery

**1.200   The following structures are normally encountered during
            dissection for a right hemicolectomy**

❑   A   caudate lobe of the liver
❑   B   inferior vena cava
❑   C   third part of the duodenum
❑   D   right ureter
❑   E   gonadal vessels

1.201   The eustachian tube

❑   A   drains the inner ear
❑   B   pierces the pharyngobasilar fascia
❑   C   gives attachment to the tensor veli palatini muscle
❑   D   can be obstructed by an enlarging palatine tonsil
❑   E   closes during swallowing

1.202   The facial nerve supplies the

❑   A   stapedius
❑   B   buccinator
❑   C   medial pterygoid
❑   D   parasympathetics to the lacrimal gland
❑   E   parasympathetics to the parotid gland

1.203   Regarding joints

❏ A   primary cartilaginous joints unite the bones of the vault of the skull at the sutures
❏ B   fibrous joints are very mobile
❏ C   symphysis pubis is an example of a secondary cartilaginous joint
❏ D   synovial joints have a capsule enclosing the joint cavity
❏ E   the cartilaginous epiphysis is a highly vascular structure

1.204   In the knee joint

❏ A   the cruciate ligaments are extracapsular
❏ B   the meniscofemoral ligament attaches to the lateral meniscus
❏ C   the oblique popliteal ligament is derived from semimembranosus insertion
❏ D   the anterior cruciate ligament prevents the femur from sliding forwards off the tibial plateau
❏ E   the suprapatellar bursa communicates with the joint

1.205   After lateral hemisection of the L5 segment of the spinal cord there is an ipsilateral

❏ A   loss of pain in the foot
❏ B   loss of fine touch in the foot
❏ C   loss of ankle jerk
❏ D   wasting of the quadriceps muscle
❏ E   Babinski sign

1.206   Lateral swellings of the neck include

❏ A   cervical ribs
❏ B   thyroglossal cysts
❏ C   pharyngeal pouches
❏ D   carotid body tumours (chemodectomas)
❏ E   laryngoceles

1.207   Midline swellings of the neck include

❏ A   cystic hygromas
❏ B   plunging ranulae
❏ C   subhyoid bursae
❏ D   branchial cysts
❏ E   arteriovenous fistulae

SECTION 2: PHYSIOLOGY – QUESTIONS

2.1   During exercise

- ❏ A   cardiac output can increase sixfold
- ❏ B   there is a decrease in Pao_2 and $Paco_2$
- ❏ C   anticipation of exercise can cause an increase in respiratory rate
- ❏ D   an increase in systolic and diastolic blood pressure is seen
- ❏ E   renal blood flow is increased
- ❏ F   there is a decrease in negative intrathoracic pressure

2.2   In strenuous exercise the following may occur

- ❏ A   increased stroke volume
- ❏ B   rise in $Paco_2$
- ❏ C   rise in blood pressure
- ❏ D   tachycardia
- ❏ E   rise in mixed venous blood O_2 saturation

2.3   The following are associated with the acute response to injury

- ❏ A   increased plasma catecholamines
- ❏ B   increased liver glycogen levels
- ❏ C   reduced insulin levels
- ❏ D   relative hypoglycaemia
- ❏ E   raised plasma fatty acids

2.4   The following cells can regenerate

- ❏ A   cardiac muscle cells
- ❏ B   peripheral nerve cells
- ❏ C   Schwann cells
- ❏ D   mucosal cells
- ❏ E   renal tubular cells

2.5   In a healthy adult man weighing 70 kg

- ❏ A   the body water content is 75%
- ❏ B   the plasma volume is approximately 5 litres
- ❏ C   approximately 1.5 litres of water are lost daily from the lungs
- ❏ D   the intracellular fluid volume is approximately two-thirds of the total body water
- ❏ E   the daily potassium requirement is approximately 3.5–5.0 mmol/kg

2.6 Wound healing

❏ A type I collagen predominates in the early stages of wound healing
❏ B epithelial regeneration occurs to cover the surface
❏ C tensile strength is associated with collagen content
❏ D collagen undergoes remodelling at the end of the first week
❏ E is unaffected by radiotherapy

2.7 In wound healing

❏ A sutured surgical wounds heal by secondary intention
❏ B fibroblasts are responsible for wound contraction
❏ C copper deficiency delays wound healing
❏ D hyperbaric oxygen significantly accelerates wound healing
❏ E healing is delayed by azathioprine

2.8 Hypertrophy involves an

❏ A increase in tissue size
❏ B increase in cell size
❏ C increase in cell number
❏ D increase in the number of mitoses

2.9 The glomerular filtration rate (GFR)

❏ A declines with age
❏ B may be measured with inulin clearance
❏ C may be estimated by creatinine clearance
❏ D is unaffected by a protein-rich meal
❏ E decreases during pregnancy

2.10 Concerning wound healing

❏ A most skin wounds regain their pre-injury strength with time
❏ B wound strength returns to 80% of pre-injury strength by 3 months in uncomplicated cases
❏ C the small bowel regains most of its strength by 10 days
❏ D type III collagen is stronger than type I collagen
❏ E there is a lag phase lasting 6 weeks following injury

2.11   During fracture healing

❏   A   a vascular pannus is formed initially at the fracture site
❏   B   bone necrosis becomes apparent after 24–48 hours
❏   C   osteoclasts lay down seams of uncalcified new bone
❏   D   the provisional callus is made up of woven bone
❏   E   woven bone is finally replaced with lamellar bone

2.12   Myocardial blood flow

❏   A   is approximately 250 ml/min at rest
❏   B   is increased by pain
❏   C   the right coronary artery typically supplies a third of the blood to the left ventricular muscle
❏   D   is dependent on arterial pressure
❏   E   occurs during systole

2.13   The pathophysiological effects of intermittent positive-pressure ventilation (IPPV) include

❏   A   reduced splanchnic blood flow
❏   B   decreased cardiac output
❏   C   hepatic failure
❏   D   hypotension
❏   E   pneumothorax
❏   F   lowered intracranial pressure

2.14   The cardiac index is defined as

❏   A   cardiac output/body surface area
❏   B   stroke volume × heart rate
❏   C   mean arterial pressure × systemic vascular resistance
❏   D   cardiac output/body weight
❏   E   cardiac output/heart rate

2.15   The heart rate

❏   A   decreases on inspiration
❏   B   increases with pressure on the eyeball
❏   C   decreases with sleep
❏   D   increases after a meal
❏   E   decreases with pressure on the sinoatrial (SA) node

2.16   Pulmonary functional residual capacity (FRC) is

❏   A   equal to vital capacity minus the maximum inspiratory capacity
❏   B   measured by the helium dilution technique
❏   C   decreased in asthma
❏   D   decreased in emphysema
❏   E   decreased in pulmonary fibrosis

2.17   A high jugular venous pressure (JVP) is associated with

❏   A   fluid overload
❏   B   pericardial effusion
❏   C   congestive cardiac failure
❏   D   pulmonary hypertension
❏   E   superior vena cava (SVC) obstruction

2.18   Functional residual capacity (FRC)

❏   A   is increased in the elderly
❏   B   represents approximately < 50% of vital capacity
❏   C   falls following abdominal surgery
❏   D   is the sum of the residual volume and expiratory reserve volume
❏   E   is increased in fibrosing alveolitis

2.19   The following actions may have a direct positive inotropic effect on the heart

❏   A   isoprenaline infusion
❏   B   GTN infusion
❏   C   intravenous calcium
❏   D   intravenous furosemide (frusemide)
❏   E   digoxin

2.20   The following cause an increase in the heart rate

❏   A   complete cardiac denervation
❏   B   intravenous adenosine
❏   C   intravenous adrenaline (epinephrine)
❏   D   salbutamol
❏   E   metronidazole

2.21   Angiotensin II

❏   A   stimulates renin release
❏   B   inhibits aldosterone release
❏   C   is a weak arteriolar vasoconstrictor
❏   D   is converted from angiotensin I in the lung
❏   E   is released in hypovolaemia

2.22   Physiological responses to a loss of circulating blood volume include

❏   A   peripheral venular vasoconstriction
❏   B   peripheral arteriolar vasoconstriction
❏   C   reduced resistance to blood flow
❏   D   transcapillary refilling
❏   E   haemoconcentration
❏   F   tachycardia

2.23   Central venous pressure (CVP)

❏   A   is affected by the Valsalva manoeuvre
❏   B   is elevated in right ventricular failure
❏   C   is normal in septic shock
❏   D   accurately reflects cardiac output
❏   E   is raised in hypertension

2.24   The oxygen–haemoglobin dissociation curve is displaced to the left by

❏   A   an increase in pH
❏   B   anaemia
❏   C   a fall in P_{CO_2}
❏   D   pyrexia
❏   E   a fall in 2,3-DPG

2.25   Regarding shock

❏   A   septic shock produces a high systemic vascular resistance (SVR) and high cardiac output (CO)
❏   B   cardiogenic shock produces a low SVR and low CO
❏   C   neurogenic shock produces a low SVR and high CO
❏   D   anaphylactic shock produces a very low lactic acid level
❏   E   septic shock produces a low SVR and high CO

2.26   Cardiopulmonary bypass

❏ A   may produce mild postoperative neuropsychological problems
❏ B   is a recognised cause of pancreatitis
❏ C   is complicated by a severe stroke in 10% of cases
❏ D   causes a thrombocythaemia
❏ E   produces elevated cortisol levels

2.27   The following factors increase cardiac output

❏ A   standing from a lying position
❏ B   eating
❏ C   rapid arrhythmias
❏ D   long-term acclimatisation at altitude
❏ E   late pregnancy
❏ F   histamine

2.28   The functional residual capacity (FRC)

❏ A   can be measured using the helium dilution technique
❏ B   is the tidal volume plus the expiratory reserve volume
❏ C   is approximately 60% of vital capacity
❏ D   is decreased when someone is supine
❏ E   is approximately 2.5 litres in a healthy adult man

2.29   Lung spirometry is able to measure

❏ A   total lung capacity
❏ B FEV_1
❏ C   residual volume
❏ D   the FEV_1:FVC ratio
❏ E   the peak expiratory flow rate

2.30   Pulse oximetry

❏ A   provides a direct indication of arterial Po_2
❏ B   has a linear relationship with oxygen carriage
❏ C   is inaccurate in the presence of high levels of carbon monoxide
❏ D   indicates adequate tissue oxygen delivery if readings are > 95%
❏ E   indicates adequate ventilation if readings are > 95%

2.31   In statistical analysis

❏   A   a type I error is finding results that are not statistically significant when the populations are identical

❏   B   a type II error is finding a statistically significant result when the populations are identical

❏   C   an unpaired *t*-test compares two groups on the assumption that the two populations are normally distributed

❏   D   parametric tests are used when data from population groups do not follow a Gaussian distribution

❏   E   non-parametric tests are less powerful than parametric tests

2.32   In statistical analysis

❏   A   the mean of a set of values is the same as the standard error

❏   B   the median of a set of values is the same as the average

❏   C   standard deviation is a measure of the variability of a set of values

❏   D   parametric tests are used for the assessment of data that follows a non-Gaussian distribution

❏   E   the outcome of a rank or score (such as Ranson's score) cannot be Gaussian in distribution

2.33   Coronary perfusion is decreased

❏   A   in hypoxia

❏   B   by ADH

❏   C   by α stimulation

❏   D   by β stimulation

2.34   **In the cardiac cycle**

❑   A   the 'a' wave of the high jugular venous pressure (JVP) corresponds to the closure of the tricuspid valve

❑   B   all the ventricles and atria are relaxed together at some time in the cardiac cycle

❑   C   the 'a–c' interval of the JVP corresponds to the PR interval on the ECG

❑   D   the descent of the 'v' wave corresponds to the opening of the mitral valve

❑   E   the first heart sound corresponds to the opening of the mitral and tricuspid valves

❑   F   the second heart sound corresponds to aortic valve closure

❑   G   isovolumetric relaxation (isometric) occurs after aortic and pulmonary valve closure

❑   H   the QRS complex commences with the first heart sound

❑   I   myocardial cells all contract at the same time

2.35   **The following can be measured (directly or indirectly) using Swan–Ganz catheterisation**

❑   A   cardiac index

❑   B FIO_2

❑   C   left ventricular stroke work

❑   D   end-tidal CO_2

❑   E   pulmonary artery occlusion pressure

2.36   **Which of the following statistical tests are examples of parametric tests**

❑   A   paired *t*-test

❑   B   unpaired *t*-test

❑   C   Wilcoxon test

❑   D   Mann–Whitney test

❑   E   ANOVA test

2.37 **The following block transmission in postsynaptic autonomic fibres**

- ❏ A suxamethonium
- ❏ B hexamethonium
- ❏ C bupivacaine
- ❏ D guanethidine
- ❏ E pentazocine
- ❏ F fentanyl

2.38 **Wound healing by secondary intention occurs**

- ❏ A when the wound edges are opposed
- ❏ B when the wound breaks apart
- ❏ C when there is irreparable skin loss
- ❏ D at the same rate as healing by primary intention
- ❏ E when the wound becomes infected

2.39 **With respect to inotropic agents**

- ❏ A adrenaline (epinephrine) stimulates α and β receptors
- ❏ B noradrenaline (norepinephrine) is predominantly a β agonist
- ❏ C dopexamine is a splanchnic vasodilator
- ❏ D dobutamine increases systemic vascular resistance
- ❏ E adrenaline may reduce renal blood flow at higher doses

2.40 **The oxygen–haemoglobin dissociation curve**

- ❏ A produces a left shift in metabolic acidosis
- ❏ B produces a right shift with an increase in red cell 2,3-DPG
- ❏ C produces a right shift with a pyrexia
- ❏ D produces a left shift with hypercarbia
- ❏ E produces a left shift with hypocapnia

2.41 **Pulmonary artery occlusion pressure (PAOP)**

- ❏ A may be used to exclude pulmonary oedema
- ❏ B is low in cardiogenic shock
- ❏ C may be useful for an aortic aneurysm repair
- ❏ D is used routinely in the management of postoperative myocardial infarction (MI)

2.42   The character of the jugular venous pressure (JVP) wave

❏   A   'a' wave refers to atrial contraction
❏   B   'c' wave refers to closure of the mitral and tricuspid valves
❏   C   'v' wave refers to a full atrium
❏   D   'v' wave occurs with and just after the carotid pulse
❏   E   'a' wave is absent in atrial fibrillation

2.43   Cerebrospinal fluid (CSF)

❏   A   has the same pH as blood
❏   B   has pressures normally lying between 20 and 25 cmH$_2$O in the supine position
❏   C   contains less glucose than blood
❏   D   contains less protein than blood
❏   E   contains less glucose than nasal mucus

2.44   In calcium homeostasis

❏   A   calcitonin reduces renal excretion
❏   B   calcitonin increases bone resorption
❏   C   vitamin D is converted to 25-hydroxycholecalciferol in the kidney
❏   D   vitamin D activation is increased by parathyroid hormone (PTH)
❏   E   oestrogen increases calcium absorption

2.45   The salivary glands

❏   A   secrete > 1000 ml/day
❏   B   produce saliva, which has about the same pH as plasma
❏   C   secrete amylase
❏   D   produce secretions that contain a higher molar concentration of potassium than that found in plasma
❏   E   produce hypertonic secretions

2.46   Neonates

❏   A   can concentrate urine to l400 mOsm/l
❏   B   weighing 3 kg have a blood volume of 450 ml
❏   C   should be operated on in theatres with an ambient temperature of 20 °C
❏   D   are often unable to tolerate oral feeds following major bowel surgery
❏   E   are recommended to have an oral feed of 350 ml/kg/day in the first week of life

2.47   Prolactin

❏   A   secretion decreases after surgery
❏   B   is under dopaminergic control
❏   C   secretion increases after trauma
❏   D   is involved in the secretion of milk during lactation
❏   E   secretion is under hypothalamic control

2.48   Insulin

❏   A   inhibits gluconeogenesis
❏   B   increases protein synthesis
❏   C   inhibits potassium entry into cells
❏   D   is synthesised by C cells of the pancreas
❏   E   increases glucose uptake by the brain

2.49   The normal function of the colon is in the absorption of

❏   A   water
❏   B   sodium
❏   C   chloride
❏   D   bicarbonate
❏   E   bile salts

2.50   Resection of the terminal ileum is associated with malabsorption of

❏   A   calcium
❏   B   vitamin B_{12}
❏   C   folic acid
❏   D   cholesterol
❏   E   bile salts

2.51 **The following may be seen in the blood film of a postsplenectomy patient**

❏ A target cells
❏ B punctate basophilia
❏ C Howell–Jolly bodies
❏ D sideroblasts
❏ E rouleaux formation

2.52 **Pancreatic secretion**

❏ A has pH > 8
❏ B contains lipase
❏ C contains enterokinase
❏ D is typically < 200 ml/day

2.53 **Triglycerides**

❏ A stimulate the secretion of pancreatic enzymes
❏ B stimulate insulin secretion
❏ C digestion by pancreatic lipase only becomes active in the presence of a cofactor
❏ D are hydrolysed into free fatty acids and phospholipids
❏ E digestion commences with lipase secretion at the base of the tongue.

2.54 **Bile salts**

❏ A may be released by cholecystokinin
❏ B decrease bowel motility
❏ C increase fat absorption
❏ D undergo enterohepatic circulation
❏ E are mainly absorbed in the proximal ileum

2.55   Chronic alcohol abuse may present with

❑   A   Wernicke's encephalopathy
❑   B   Korsakoff's syndrome
❑   C   cerebellar ataxia
❑   D   impotence
❑   E   Sydenham's chorea
❑   F   lymphopenia
❑   G   macrocytosis
❑   H   menorrhagia

2.56   The colon can

❑   A   absorb up to 5 litres of water a day
❑   B   produce short-chain fatty acids from cellulose
❑   C   go into ileus following a laparotomy
❑   D   exchange chloride and bicarbonate ions

2.57   A term infant weighing 3.1 kg

❑   A   requires about 450 ml of formula milk daily for adequate fluid
         and calories
❑   B   should be maintained on 700 ml of normal saline per day
         intravenously
❑   C   is at high risk of necrotising enterocolitis
❑   D   is at risk of developing hypoglycaemia postoperatively
❑   E   should pass meconium in the first 24 hours after birth

2.58   Potassium

❑   A   is raised in metabolic alkalosis
❑   B   concentration in plasma is low in chronic adrenal insufficiency
❑   C   loss may cause renal tubular damage
❑   D   is the main intracellular cation
❑   E   level in plasma is a reliable index of total body potassium

2.59 **The following may have a lower potassium concentration than plasma**

❑ A saliva
❑ B ileostomy fluid
❑ C sweat
❑ D cerebrospinal fluid (CSF)
❑ E gastric juice

2.60 **The following would lower the plasma potassium concentration**

❑ A extracellular fluid depletion
❑ B severe diarrhoea
❑ C metabolic alkalosis
❑ D hyperaldosteronism
❑ E acute tubular necrosis

2.61 **Prolonged vomiting due to pyloric stenosis would cause**

❑ A a rise in serum urea
❑ B a rise in standard bicarbonate
❑ C hyperkalaemia
❑ D hyperchloraemia
❑ E a rise in arterial P_{CO_2}

2.62 **Extracellular fluid differs from intracellular fluid by having a**

❑ A higher chloride concentration
❑ B lower potassium concentration
❑ C greater volume
❑ D lower protein concentration
❑ E lower pH

2.63 **Plasma volume can be measured by using**

❑ A urea
❑ B deuterium
❑ C inulin
❑ D iodinated serum albumin
❑ E Evans blue

2.64   Renal blood flow

❑   A   is related to blood volume
❑   B   can be estimated by para-aminohippuric acid (PAH) clearance
❑   C   increases in hypovolaemic shock
❑   D   is related to the plasma concentration of antidiuretic hormone (ADH)
❑   E   decreases in hypercarbia

2.65   In the loop of Henle

❑   A   water moves out of the descending limb into the interstitium
❑   B   the descending limb is impermeable to urea
❑   C   chloride is transported from the tubular fluid into the ascending limb
❑   D   the high osmolality maintains the counter-current mechanism
❑   E   sodium concentration decreases as the descending limb travels downwards

2.66   Renin

❑   A   is secreted in response to a reduced renal blood flow
❑   B   is produced by the macula densa
❑   C   is increased immediately after surgery
❑   D   is secreted in response to low oxygen tension in the renal artery
❑   E   is responsible for the conversion of angiotensin I to angiotensin II

2.67   In dehydration

❑   A   renal blood flow will increase
❑   B   urine output may decrease to 600 ml/24 h
❑   C   approximately 85% of the glomerular filtrate is reabsorbed in the proximal renal tubule
❑   D   interstitial fluid in the medulla of the kidney is hypertonic
❑   E   fluid in the distal convoluted tubule is hypertonic with respect to plasma

2.68 **Release of oxygen from the blood to peripheral tissues is influenced by**

❏ A temperature
❏ B pH
❏ C blood volume
❏ D P_{CO_2}
❏ E osmotic pressure

2.69 **Carbon dioxide**

❏ A is carried predominantly as bicarbonate (HCO_3^-)
❏ B is mainly dissolved in plasma
❏ C is more soluble than oxygen
❏ D causes systemic vasodilatation
❏ E diffuses with difficulty into red blood cells

2.70 **Lung compliance is reduced by**

❏ A a decrease in the elastic fibres in the lung parenchyma
❏ B an increase in the surface tension of the alveolar fluid
❏ C pulmonary contusion
❏ D an open pneumothorax
❏ E an increase in functional residual capacity

2.71 **Stimulation of arterial chemoreceptors by hypoxaemia may result in**

❏ A respiratory depression
❏ B respiratory alkalosis
❏ C increase in arterial blood pressure
❏ D increased blood flow to the brain
❏ E increased blood flow to skeletal muscles

2.72 **Increased pulmonary ventilation is stimulated by**

❏ A increased arterial P_{CO_2}
❏ B decreased pH
❏ C decreased arterial P_{O_2}
❏ D reflex activation in the respiratory centre in the cerebellum
❏ E carotid body chemoreceptors

2.73 A tracheostomy will

❏ A reduce airway resistance
❏ B reduce residual volume
❏ C reduce vital capacity
❏ D reduce physiological dead space
❏ E increase lung compliance

2.74 Following major abdominal surgery, there is a

❏ A decrease in tidal volume
❏ B decreased minute ventilatory volume
❏ C decrease in functional residual capacity
❏ D increase in anatomical dead space
❏ E decrease in lung compliance

2.75 Carotid baroreceptors are stimulated by

❏ A increased arterial P_{CO_2}
❏ B fall in arterial P_{CO_2}
❏ C anaemia
❏ D rise in pulse pressure
❏ E rise in mean arterial pressure

2.76 The carotid body is stimulated by

❏ A a fall in metabolic rate
❏ B a rise in blood pH
❏ C a fall in arterial P_{O_2}
❏ D an increase in arterial P_{CO_2}
❏ E a fall in arterial P_{CO_2}

2.77 During exercise increased cardiac output is associated with

❏ A raised central venous pressure (CVP)
❏ B a decrease in end-systolic volume
❏ C a small increase in end-diastolic volume
❏ D increased stroke volume
❏ E increased myocardial contractility

2.78   Cerebral blood flow is increased by

❏   A   a rise in body temperature
❏   B   an increase in Po_2
❏   C   an increase in arterial Pco_2
❏   D   raised intracranial pressure
❏   E   noradrenaline (norepinephrine)

2.79   Blood flow in muscle is influenced by

❏   A   sympathetic stimulation
❏   B   bradykinin
❏   C   parasympathetic stimulation
❏   D   arterial blood pressure
❏   E   temperature

2.80   Hypovolaemic shock

❏   A   causes increased cerebral perfusion
❏   B   produces a raised central venous pressure (CVP)
❏   C   reduces skin perfusion
❏   D   leads to a fall in renal blood flow
❏   E   is associated with a normal cardiac output

2.81   Secretin

❏   A   inhibits gallbladder contraction
❏   B   stimulates secretion of alkaline pancreatic juice
❏   C   is secreted by the stomach
❏   D   stimulates enzyme-rich secretion from the pancreas
❏   E   secretion is stimulated by acid from the duodenum

2.82   Fat absorption is facilitated by

❏   A   bile pigments
❏   B   bile salts
❏   C   vitamin D
❏   D   carbohydrate
❏   E   lipase

2.83   The colon is involved in the absorption of

❑   A   sodium
❑   B   chloride
❑   C   bicarbonate
❑   D   bile salts
❑   E   amino acids

2.84   A total gastrectomy may lead to malabsorption of

❑   A   iron
❑   B   vitamin B_{12}
❑   C   vitamin D
❑   D   glucose
❑   E   vitamin C

2.85   High levels of circulating adrenaline (epinephrine) will produce

❑   A   lycosuria
❑   B   excessive sweating
❑   C   bradycardia
❑   D   paroxysmal hypotension
❑   E   bronchospasm

2.86   Intravenous infusion of adrenaline (epinephrine) would cause

❑   A   an increase in heart rate
❑   B   increased gut peristalsis
❑   C   a decrease in splanchnic blood flow
❑   D   bronchodilatation
❑   E   pupillary constriction

2.87   Prolonged elevation of plasma cortisol would result in

❑   A   osteoporosis
❑   B   increased protein catabolism
❑   C   hyperglycaemia
❑   D   a fall in plasma albumin
❑   E   a lowering of the serum potassium

2.88 **The following hormones are not under the influence of the pituitary gland**

- ❑ A calcitonin
- ❑ B aldosterone
- ❑ C thyroid stimulating hormone
- ❑ D growth hormone
- ❑ E parathyroid hormone

2.89 **In the central nervous system**

- ❑ A pain is perceived in the thalamus
- ❑ B the left motor cortex controls the right side of the body
- ❑ C proprioception is conveyed in the posterior columns
- ❑ D spinal reflex activity can be modulated by descending spinal pathways
- ❑ E neurones conveying thermal sensation rarely cross to the contralateral spinal cord

2.90 **Sodium depletion could cause**

- ❑ A muscle weakness
- ❑ B tachycardia
- ❑ C raised blood pressure
- ❑ D reduced cardiac output
- ❑ E decreased body weight

2.91 **The distal convoluted tubule is the site of**

- ❑ A potassium secretion
- ❑ B hydrogen ion secretion
- ❑ C aldosterone-regulated reabsorption of sodium
- ❑ D principal water reabsorption in the kidney
- ❑ E the action of antidiuretic hormone (ADH)

2.92 **Hypothermia**

- ❑ A increases blood viscosity
- ❑ B prolongs the clotting time of blood
- ❑ C increases the oxygen content of blood at any given tension
- ❑ D would cause cardiac arrest below 25 °C
- ❑ E has few effects on the heart

2.93   Direct energy sources for the brain include

❑   A   products of aerobic glycolysis
❑   B   ketone bodies
❑   C   amino acids
❑   D   fat
❑   E   lactic acid

2.94   Glycogenesis in the liver is stimulated by

❑   A   glucagon
❑   B   insulin
❑   C   cortisol
❑   D   adrenaline (epinephrine)
❑   E   thyroxine

2.95   Hypomagnesaemia

❑   A   produces similar clinical effects to hypocalcaemia
❑   B   is associated with muscle weakness
❑   C   is associated with small bowel resection
❑   D   in the plasma is a good indicator of total body magnesium
❑   E   has to be corrected by infusion only

2.96   Metabolic rate

❑   A   is lower in children than adults
❑   B   is affected by surface area
❑   C   falls after a meal
❑   D   falls in a cold environment

2.97   The body's acute response to injury includes

❑   A   an increase in the visceral blood flow
❑   B   a fall in plasma insulin concentration during the ebb phase of injury
❑   C   an increase in hepatic glycogenolysis and gluconeogenesis
❑   D   stimulation of aldosterone secretion, leading to metabolic alkalosis
❑   E   a rise in serum albumin

2.98   Concerning gangrene

❏ A   in established gangrene, sensation is preserved in the affected part
❏ B   dry gangrene occurs when both venous and arterial obstruction are present
❏ C   diabetic gangrene of the toes can occur in the presence of normal foot pulses
❏ D   gas gangrene is usually painless
❏ E   synergistic spreading gangrene can be successfully treated with intravenous antibiotics

2.99   Raised intracranial pressure

❏ A   can be caused by shearing injury to the scalp
❏ B   occurs immediately after an acute subdural haematoma
❏ C   leads to a rise in cerebral perfusion pressure
❏ D   causes dilatation of the ipsilateral pupil
❏ E   can lead to a rise in blood pressure and a bradycardia

2.100   In wound healing

❏ A   platelets help in initiating the inflammatory response during acute wound healing
❏ B   monocytes are more abundant than neutrophils during the later stages of healing
❏ C   protease levels are increased in chronic wounds
❏ D   hypertrophic scars extend beyond the margins of the original scar
❏ E   keloids usually develop within 2–3 weeks of initial injury

2.101   In the liver

❏ A   unconjugated bilirubin is water-insoluble
❏ B   urinary urobilinogen levels are increased in prehepatic jaundice
❏ C   dark urine and pale stools are classical features of post-hepatic jaundice
❏ D   pruritis is seen only in hepatic cholestasis
❏ E   stones in the common bile duct usually lead to a dilated gallbladder

2.102 Bacterial flexor tenosynovitis

❑ A commonly affects the thumb or ring finger
❑ B is usually caused by *Staphylococcus aureus* infection
❑ C does not affect the movements of the digit
❑ D causes destruction of synovial gliding surfaces
❑ E can lead to permanent tendon damage

2.103 Saliva

❑ A flow rate increases during nausea
❑ B secreted from the submandibular gland is predominantly mucous in nature
❑ C volume production approaches 1 litre a day
❑ D secretion ceases at night
❑ E contains only a low concentration of potassium

2.104 Regarding thyroid gland physiology

❑ A greater amounts of tri-iodothyronine (T3) are secreted than thyroxine (T4)
❑ B iodine is transported into the gland along a concentration gradient
❑ C tri-iodothyronine (T3) is mainly bound to albumin in plasma
❑ D thyroxine-binding globulin is produced in the liver
❑ E thyroxine has a half-life of approximately 24 hours

2.105 Insulin

❑ A permits glucose transport against a concentration gradient
❑ B enhances glucose transport across the cell membrane
❑ C enhances glucose transport across renal tubular epithelium
❑ D has no effect on glucose transport into the brain
❑ E enhances glucose transport across the intestinal mucosa

2.106 Thyroxine

❑ A increases the oxygen consumption rate
❑ B decreases the rate of muscle synthesis
❑ C decreases the plasma concentration of cholesterol
❑ D decreases lipolysis

2.107 Cereberospinal fluid (CSF)

❑   A   is absorbed by the choroid plexus
❑   B   absorption is dependent on CSF pressure
❑   C   has a lower glucose concentration than plasma
❑   D   has an equal protein concentration to that of plasma

2.108 Aldosterone acts on the renal tubules to

❑   A   increase excretion of magnesium
❑   B   decrease secretion of hydrogen
❑   C   decrease reabsorption of sodium
❑   D   increase secretion of potassium
❑   E   decrease excretion of ammonium

2.109 Macrophages

❑   A   are derived from the bone marrow
❑   B   have phagocytic properties
❑   C   are important in humoral immunity
❑   D   can form megaloblasts
❑   E   are characteristically found in granulomas

2.110 General host factors predisposing to wound infection include

❑   A   hypoxia
❑   B   pyrexia
❑   C   jaundice
❑   D   hypercalcaemia
❑   E   anaemia

2.111 Signs of increased intracranial pressure include

❑   A   increased pulse rate
❑   B   increased blood pressure
❑   C   neck stiffness
❑   D   bloody tap following lumbar puncture
❑   E   respiratory depression

2.112 Inflammation is characterised by

- ❏ A increased blood flow
- ❏ B decreased vascular permeability
- ❏ C recruitment of cells that phagocytose microbes and damaged tissue
- ❏ D secretion of preformed mediators
- ❏ E an inflammatory response that is independent of the burden of tissue injury

2.113 In the cell cycle

- ❏ A RNA and proteins are synthesised during the G1 phase
- ❏ B duplication of cellular DNA occurs during the G2 phase
- ❏ C the average duration of the cell cycle is approximately 10 days
- ❏ D mitosis occurs during the M phase
- ❏ E tumour growth follows Gompertzian kinetics
- ❏ F cytotoxic drugs act mainly on resting cells

2.114 Renal blood flow

- ❏ A may be reduced by 50% in acute renal failure
- ❏ B is normally kept constant by autoregulation
- ❏ C is higher in the medulla than in the cortex
- ❏ D is unaffected by hypertension

2.115 The intramural pH of the stomach

- ❏ A is calculated using the Henderson–Hasselbalch equation
- ❏ B is considered normal if pH = 7.2
- ❏ C is dependent on the luminal bicarbonate concentration being equivalent to the plasma bicarbonate concentration
- ❏ D is increased in a state of metabolic acidosis
- ❏ E is decreased in profound hypovolaemia

2.116 Nitric oxide

- ❏ A causes platelet aggregation
- ❏ B causes relaxation of smooth muscle
- ❏ C uptake is increased by endotoxins
- ❏ D diffuses freely between cells
- ❏ E causes vasodilatation

2.117   Monopolar surgical diathermy

❑   A   uses an alternating current of 400 Hz
❑   B   requires a patient plate electrode of at least 20 cm²
❑   C   may be used for 'cutting' tissue
❑   D   may be safely applied through ordinary surgical forceps
❑   E   produces a local heating effect up to 1000 °C
❑   F   is safer than bipolar diathermy
❑   G   should not be used in patients with pacemakers
❑   H   produces burn injuries that are usually partial thickness

2.118   Nutritional status may be estimated from

❑   A   triceps muscle circumference
❑   B   body mass index
❑   C   serum lymphocyte transferrin
❑   D   hand-grip strength
❑   E   serum albumin

2.119   In metabolic acidosis

❑   A   there is a negative base excess
❑   B   bicarbonate is the main intracellular buffer
❑   C   proteins and phosphates are the main extracellular buffer
❑   D   compensation occurs by an increase in alveolar ventilation
❑   E   bicarbonate infusion is the mainstay of treatment

2.120   Complications of total parenteral nutrition (TPN) include

❑   A   hypocalcaemia
❑   B   hypercalcaemia
❑   C   hypokalaemia
❑   D   hypophosphataemia
❑   E   hyperuricaemia

2.121   Potential sequelae of terminal ileal resection include

❑   A   vitamin B$_{12}$ deficiency
❑   B   folic acid deficiency
❑   C   iron deficiency
❑   D   gallstones
❑   E   pernicious anaemia
❑   F   diarrhoea

2.122   A 200-ml bolus of Gelofusine®

❏   A   produces a sustained (5-minutes) rise of 2 cmH_2O in a
             dehydrated patient
❏   B   produces an initial rise and fall in central venous pressure (CVP)
             in a dehydrated patient
❏   C   can produce the same intravascular expansion as 1 litre of
             normal saline
❏   D   producing a sustained CVP rise of more than 4 cmH_2O may
             indicate overfilling
❏   E   may produce anaphylactic shock

2.123   A 5% dextrose intravenous infusion

❏   A   is isotonic on administration
❏   B   remains within the extracellular intravascular space for at least
             1 hour
❏   C   is a good mode of resuscitation in the shocked patient
❏   D   may give rise to type II respiratory failure
❏   E   contains 60 kcal/l (~251 J)

2.124   Metabolic acidosis is seen in

❏   A   vomiting
❏   B   hyperaldosteronism
❏   C   diabetic ketoacidosis
❏   D   renal failure
❏   E   hyperparathyroidism
❏   F   septic shock

2.125   Respiratory acidosis may be seen in

❏   A   pneumonia
❏   B   crushing chest injury
❏   C   excessive mechanical ventilation
❏   D   pulmonary embolus (small)
❏   E   head injury
❏   F   tracheostomy

2.126   Hyperbaric oxygen therapy

❑   A   can be used in the treatment of carbon monoxide poisoning
❑   B   can be administered using an anaesthetic breathing circuit
❑   C   may cause acute oxygen toxicity
❑   D   requires the use of a pressurised chamber
❑   E   typically consists of one 20-minute session

2.127   Haemorrhage

❑   A   is defined as an acute or chronic loss of circulating blood
❑   B   the normal adult blood volume is approximately 5% of body weight
❑   C   the blood volume of obese patients is estimated using their ideal body weight
❑   D   the blood volume of children is approximately 15% of their body weight
❑   E   tachycardia is the earliest measurable sign

2.128   Common causes of a pulseless electrical activity (PEA) arrest include

❑   A   hypovolaemia
❑   B   electric shock
❑   C   tension pneumothorax
❑   D   hypoxia
❑   E   cardiac tamponade

2.129   In respiratory alkalosis

❑   A   carpopedal spasm may be corrected by rebreathing into a bag
❑   B   tetany occurs due to changes in calcium–protein binding
❑   C   there is a lowering of the plasma carbonic acid concentration
❑   D   there is an elevated bicarbonate concentration in plasma
❑   E   the P_{CO_2} is < 5 kPa

2.130   In the heart, the right ventricle

❑   A   is the most likely chamber to be injured in a stabbing
❑   B   is the most anterior heart chamber
❑   C   is best visualised by transoesophageal echocardiography
❑   D   is supplied by the right coronary artery
❑   E   receives no blood from the lungs

2.131 **In the immediate postoperative period following an anterior resection there is increased**

❏ A urinary sodium loss
❏ B secretion of ADH
❏ C urea production
❏ D urine osmolality
❏ E glomerular filtration rate

2.132 **Heat loss during laparotomy may be minimised by**

❏ A humidification of inspired gases
❏ B lavage with warm saline
❏ C maintaining the environmental temperature at 20 °C
❏ D use of a heated blanket set at 35 °C
❏ E use of a heat-reflecting blanket

3.11 **The incidence of postoperative wound infection in abdominal surgery is increased with**

❏ A   extensive diathermy use
❏ B   not wearing masks
❏ C   inadequate haemostasis
❏ D   well-controlled diabetes mellitus
❏ E   steroid therapy
❏ F   ciclosporin treatment

3.12 **Human immunodeficiency virus (HIV)**

❏ A   has been contracted by droplet aerosol created by orthopaedic power tools
❏ B   leads to a persistently elevated antigen titre
❏ C   most frequently leads to a reversal of the CD4/CD8 lymphocyte ratio
❏ D   has a transmission rate of about 1% following percutaneous exposure
❏ E   is less infectious than hepatitis B virus

3.13 **Osteomyelitis**

❏ A   most commonly arises in adults as a result of a haematogenous infection from a primary focus elsewhere in the body
❏ B   is most commonly caused by *Escherichia coli* in neonates
❏ C   is most commonly due to *Staphylococcus* spp. in adults
❏ D   may not be apparent on X-ray for up to 14 days after the onset of symptoms
❏ E   can be treated by early high-dose intravenous antibiotics as part of the treatment regimen

3.14 **Tourniquets**

❏ A   may be applied safely for up to 3 hours at a time
❏ B   should not be applied to cause a pressure exceeding 300 mmHg
❏ C   can cause focal demyelination of peripheral nerves
❏ D   usually produce an axonotmesis
❏ E   are suitable for procedures under local anaesthesia

3.15 The Nd-YAG laser

❏ A has very little tissue penetration
❏ B is principally used for tattoo removal
❏ C has a role in the palliation of oesophageal carcinoma
❏ D should be used in a designated 'Laser Controlled Area'
❏ E requires compulsory eye protection by the user

3.16 Keloid scars

❏ A are more common in pigmented skin
❏ B occur within the limits of the surgical wound
❏ C are most common on the flexure surfaces of the limbs
❏ D may be re-excised with good results
❏ E may respond to pressure dressing
❏ F can be prevented by using subcuticular sutures

3.17 Regarding pulmonary tuberculosis

❏ A *Mycobacterium tuberculosis bovis* is the predominant cause
❏ B transmission is usually by ingestion of infected milk
❏ C there is a rising incidence in Western countries
❏ D induced hypersensitivity reaction is mediated by B lymphocytes
❏ E Gohn focus refers to involved regional lymph nodes
❏ F Gohn complex refers to the combination of the Gohn focus and involved regional lymph nodes
❏ G Gohn focus is usually subpleural in location

3.18 Actinomycosal infection

❏ A is most commonly found in the groin
❏ B is most commonly due to *Actinomyces propionibacterium*
❏ C usually produces positive cultures at 48 hours
❏ D produces a characteristic discharge containing sulphur granules
❏ E is caused by Gram-negative obligate anaerobic bacteria

3.19 Human immunodeficiency virus (HIV) infection

❏ A   is caused by a retrovirus
❏ B   may be diagnosed by Western blotting
❏ C   is present in high titre in the blood of asymptomatic carriers
❏ D   carries a risk of seroconversion following a needlestick injury from an HIV-positive patient of approximately 1 in 25
❏ E   is more infectious following a needlestick injury than hepatitis B

3.20 In hydatid disease

❏ A   the causative bacteria is *Echinococcus granulosus*
❏ B   humans are accidental intermediate hosts
❏ C   the normal intermediate host is the dog
❏ D   hepatic lesions are often asymptomatic
❏ E   diagnosis is made on needle aspiration of suspected lesions

3.21 Regarding sterilisation of surgical equipment

❏ A   chemical sterilisation is appropriate for equipment unsuitable for exposure to steam
❏ B   2% glutaraldehyde can be used for plastic equipment
❏ C   dry-heat sterilisation may be appropriate for equipment that is not well penetrated by steam

3.22 *Clostridium difficile* infection

❏ A   may be adequately treated with a single dose of oral metronidazole
❏ B   is usually diagnosed by Gram staining of the faeces
❏ C   may be adequately treated with oral vancomycin
❏ D   should be followed up by stool culture in asymptomatic patients
❏ E   may lead to colonic perforation

3.23 *Clostridium difficile* infection

❏ A   has been increasing in incidence during the past 10 years
❏ B   is only caused by antibiotic treatment
❏ C   is most commonly caused by gentamicin
❏ D   the diarrhoea typically starts within a week of commencing antibiotics
❏ E   spores may be found in dust

3.24   Actinomycosis infection

❑ A   is very sensitive to penicillin treatment
❑ B   is frequently found in association with other bacteria
❑ C   is caused by Gram-negative rods
❑ D   may mimic inflammatory bowel disease
❑ E   usually resolves with antibiotics when associated with abscess formation

3.25   In viral hepatitis

❑ A   persistence of hepatitis B surface antigen indicates an increased risk of developing chronic liver disease
❑ B   chronic hepatitis B infection increases the risk of developing gallbladder carcinoma
❑ C   hepatitis C virus accounts for about 90% of cases of post-transfusion hepatitis
❑ D   the acute illness of hepatitis C virus is generally less severe than that of hepatitis B virus infection

3.26   The risk of overwhelming postsplenectomy sepsis may be reduced by

❑ A   HiB vaccination
❑ B   hepatitis B vaccination
❑ C   poliomyelitis vaccination
❑ D   prophylactic metronidazole
❑ E   pneumococcal vaccination

3.27   *Echinococcus granulosus*

❑ A   the mature form is found in dogs
❑ B   the cyst stage is found in humans
❑ C   causes epilepsy
❑ D   causes anaphylaxis
❑ E   causes peritonitis
❑ F   carries a risk for hepatocellular carcinoma
❑ G   is a cestode (tapeworm)

3.28   In immunity and infection

❏   A   interferons are a family of glycoproteins, which are released from virally infected cells
❏   B   natural killer cells are circulating lymphocytes capable of destroying virally infected cells without prior sensitisation
❏   C   the cytotoxic activity of natural killer cells is greatly reduced by the presence of interferon
❏   D   natural killer cells have no role in the destruction of malignant cells
❏   E   adaptive immunity, unlike innate immunity, is found only in higher animals

3.29   Immunocompromised patients

❏   A   have no impairment of wound healing
❏   B   have no increased complication rate following minor surgery
❏   C   have a high incidence of anorectal sepsis with HIV infection
❏   D   should not undergo surgery for anorectal abscesses with HIV infection
❏   E   may develop pyomyositis, which may present as an abscess

3.30   Human immunodeficiency virus (HIV)

❏   A   is less infectious than hepatitis B virus
❏   B   patients should be barrier-nursed
❏   C   risk for surgeons can be decreased by vaccination
❏   D   risk for surgeons is greater with a solid than with a hollow needlestick injury
❏   E   risk is greater for pathologists than for surgeons

3.31   Organs normally colonised by commensal bacteria include the

❏   A   oropharynx
❏   B   peritoneal cavity
❏   C   lung parenchyma
❏   D   retina
❏   E   aqueous humour

3.32   Toxins produced by *Staphylococcus aureus* include

❑ A   verotoxin
❑ B   hyaluronidase
❑ C   toxic-shock syndrome toxin
❑ D   haemolysin
❑ E   enterotoxin
❑ F   collagenase

3.33   In acute inflammation, neutrophils

❑ A   actively migrate into tissues
❑ B   migrate in response to bradykinin
❑ C   migrate in response to components of complement
❑ D   have an average lifespan of 10 days in the tissues
❑ E   respond to colony-stimulating factors

3.34   In resuscitation

❑ A   gelatins may cause anaphylaxis
❑ B   colloid is adequate for intestinal fluid replacement
❑ C   it is best to use whole blood in haemorrhaging trauma cases
❑ D   Gelofusin® contains a high level of potassium
❑ E   normal saline contains 132 mmol/l of sodium

3.35   Asplenic patients are at a particularly increased risk of overwhelming sepsis from

❑ A   anaerobic bacteria
❑ B   *Streptococcus pneumoniae*
❑ C   *Neisseria meningitidis*
❑ D   *Haemophilus influenzae*
❑ E   *Bacteroides fragilis*
❑ F   fungi

3.36   The enteral route of nutrition

❑ A   may cause bacterial overgrowth in the gut
❑ B   reduces stress ulceration
❑ C   is less expensive than the parenteral route
❑ D   decreases the incidence of cholestasis by promoting biliary flow
❑ E   may be commenced immediately after gastrointestinal surgery

3.37   Postoperative hypoxaemia

❏   A   is especially common after upper abdominal surgery
❏   B   may account for some cases of postoperative confusion
❏   C   occurs episodically with regional anaesthesia
❏   D   can persist for up to 3 days postoperatively
❏   E   is less common with narcotic infusions than it is with bolus
            doses

3.38   Side effects of steroids include

❏   A   avascular necrosis of bone
❏   B   pancreatitis
❏   C   hepatotoxicity
❏   D   depression
❏   E   bone marrow suppression

3.39   Hyponatraemia may occur

❏   A   with excess steroids
❏   B   in burns
❏   C   in fever
❏   D   in renal failure
❏   E   following transurethral resection of prostate (TURP)
❏   F   in intestinal obstruction
❏   G   in pyloric stenosis

**3.40   Prolonged irrigation with glycine during a transurethral
          prostatectomy may cause**

❏   A   clotting abnormality
❏   B   coma
❏   C   hypokalaemia
❏   D   hypocalcaemia
❏   E   metabolic alkalosis

3.41   Haemolytic anaemia

❏   A   is characteristically microcytic
❏   B   may lead to gallstones
❏   C   causes elevated urine urobilinogen levels
❏   D   causes elevated serum haptoglobin levels
❏   E   is associated with a conjugated hyperbilirubinaemia

3.42   In fluid replacement for bleeding secondary to trauma

❏ A   excessive crystalloid administration is associated with adult respiratory distress syndrome (ARDS)
❏ B   initial volume expansion is more quickly achieved with crystalloid rather than colloid
❏ C   colloid administration prevents a fall in haematocrit level
❏ D   stored blood has a high pH
❏ E   blood is the fluid of choice to correct an ongoing haemorrhage and hypotension

3.43   Third-space fluid loss in the perioperative period

❏ A   is related to the degree of tissue injury
❏ B   can be up to 15 ml/kg/hour
❏ C   has a fluid composition similar to interstitial fluid
❏ D   is best replaced by dextrose-saline
❏ E   includes losses from enterocutaneous fistulae

3.44   Cytotoxic T cells

❏ A   act via specific antigen receptors
❏ B   are lymphocytes that are able to kill virally infected cells after prior sensitisation
❏ C   do not have a role in graft rejection
❏ D   play a major role in the protection of body surfaces
❏ E   are involved in atopic dermatitis

3.45   The following conditions may be associated with a microcytic anaemia

❏ A   β-thalassaemia
❏ B   carcinoma of the rectum
❏ C   hereditary haemochromatosis
❏ D   menorrhagia
❏ E   chronic renal failure

3.46   Fresh-frozen plasma (FFP)

❑ A   must be thawed on the ward or in the operating theatre
❑ B   contains albumin
❑ C   may cause a severe transfusion reaction
❑ D   contains immunoglobulins
❑ E   is the blood product of choice for replacing fibrinogen

3.47   In haemophilia

❑ A   mucosal membrane bleeding is the hallmark of haemophilia A
❑ B   female carriers of haemophilia A have no bleeding tendency
❑ C   haemophilia B is inherited as an autosomal recessive trait
❑ D   haemophilia B is a deficiency in factor IX
❑ E   pseudotumours may complicate intramuscular bleeds in patients with haemophilia A

3.48   Folate deficiency occurs in

❑ A   methotrexate therapy
❑ B   alcoholism
❑ C   pregnancy
❑ D   ileal resection
❑ E   Cushing's syndrome
❑ F   short-bowel syndrome

3.49   Deep vein thrombosis (DVT)

❑ A   occurs in 30% of surgical cases without surgical prophylaxis
❑ B   remains undetected in 50% of cases
❑ C   extends above the popliteal vein in 40% of cases
❑ D   incidence is increased in protein C deficiency
❑ E   is decreased in antithrombin III deficiency

3.50   Chronic iron deficiency anaemia

❑ A   produces a right shift of the oxygen dissociation curve
❑ B   elevates the total iron binding capacity (TIBC)
❑ C   causes a low Pco_2
❑ D   is associated with dysphagia
❑ E   can be associated with aspirin therapy

3.51   Fibrinolysis

❑   A   is augmented by epsilon-aminocaproic acid (EACA)
❑   B   is inhibited by tranexamic acid
❑   C   is associated with protein C deficiency
❑   D   tPA is the commonest activator
❑   E   may be activated by factor XII

3.52   Vitamin B$_{12}$

❑   A   is involved in the red cell maturation process
❑   B   is involved in platelet synthesis
❑   C   is stored longer than vitamin C
❑   D   is the same as intrinsic factor
❑   E   is absorbed maximally in the duodenum

3.53   The following interfere with blood cross-matching and compatibility tests

❑   A   Dextran-40
❑   B   aspirin
❑   C   clopidogrel
❑   D   warfarin
❑   E   Gelofusine®

3.54   Human albumin solution

❑   A   is the most effective agent for acute volume replacement
❑   B   may induce hyponatraemia
❑   C   is useful in managing chronic liver disease
❑   D   must be stored at 4 °C
❑   E   is subject to a virus-inactivating procedure during manufacture

3.55   Autologous transfusion of precollected blood

❑   A   carries no risk of a transfusion reaction
❑   B   is useful in patients with multiple alloantibodies
❑   C   is a safe technique in all patients
❑   D   can supply up to 10 units of blood
❑   E   is prohibited by UK guidelines for use in patients with viral hepatitis

3.56   In the coagulation cascade

❑   A   synthesis of factors II, VII, IX and X is vitamin K-dependent
❑   B   the intrinsic pathway includes factor VII
❑   C   fibrinogen cleaves prothrombin to yield thrombin
❑   D   factor VIII is synthesised mainly in the vascular endothelium
❑   E   antithrombin III deficiency predisposes to bleeding
❑   F   factor V deficiency predisposes to bleeding

3.57   Disseminated intravascular coagulation (DIC)

❑   A   may present with thrombosis
❑   B   should be considered in septic patients with a rising platelet count
❑   C   is present in patients with raised fibrin degradation products
❑   D   is associated with adenocarcinoma of the bowel
❑   E   sometimes requires fresh-frozen plasma and platelet transfusion

3.58   The treatment of acute haemolytic transfusion reaction includes

❑   A   removing the intravenous cannula from the patient
❑   B   fluid restriction to avoid pulmonary oedema
❑   C   furosemide (frusemide)
❑   D   1 litre of 20% mannitol
❑   E   insertion of a central line in an oliguric patient

3.59   The following conditions may be associated with a raised mean cell volume

❑   A   dietary iron deficiency
❑   B   vegan diet
❑   C   alcoholic liver disease
❑   D   recovery from acute haemorrhage
❑   E   chronic haemolytic anaemia

3.60   Prolongation of the activated partial thromboplastin time (APTT)

❑   A   usually occurs with low-molecular-weight heparin treatment
❑   B   occurs after warfarin treatment
❑   C   indicates adequacy of thromboprophylaxis with subcutaneous heparin
❑   D   is usual in patients receiving intravenous heparin
❑   E   may indicate a lupus anticoagulant

3.61   Petechial haemorrhages are seen in

❑   A   scurvy
❑   B   fat embolus
❑   C   vitamin K deficiency
❑   D   von Willebrand's disease

3.62   Platelet count

❑   A   of $< 50 \times 10^9/l$ is likely to result in spontaneous bleeding of the colon
❑   B   may be elevated in patients with an adenocarcinoma
❑   C   characteristically falls after splenectomy
❑   D   may be influenced by phlebotomy technique
❑   E   may be decreased in patients with an adenocarcinoma of the colon

3.63   Regarding coagulation factors

❑   A   the principal site of synthesis is the vascular endothelium
❑   B   tissue-factor expression by tumours may predispose to thrombosis
❑   C   protein C has anticoagulant activity
❑   D   protein S has anticoagulant activity
❑   E   factor VII is a component of the extrinsic pathway

3.64   Immune-mediated transfusion reactions

❑   A   must be due to ABO incompatibility if haemolysis occurs
❑   B   may be due to a secondary antibody response
❑   C   affect more than 10–20% of red cell or platelet transfusions
❑   D   may be due to plasma protein antigens
❑   E   may be due to white cell antigens

3.65   Possible complications of blood transfusion include

❑   A   graft-versus-host disease
❑   B   an increased risk of recurrent malignancy
❑   C   pancreatic endocrine insufficiency
❑   D   life-threatening thrombocytopenia
❑   E   T-cell leukaemia

3.66   The following are recognised sequelae of a massive blood transfusion

❑   A   hyperkalaemia
❑   B   hypocalcaemia
❑   C   dilutional thrombocytopenia
❑   D   adult respiratory distress syndrome (ARDS)
❑   E   hyperthermia

3.67   Cardiopulmonary bypass

❑   A   is often associated with thrombocytosis
❑   B   is often associated with platelet dysfunction
❑   C   is usually combined with induced hyperthermia
❑   D   does not affect coagulation factor levels
❑   E   needs to be followed by vitamin K administration at the end of the procedure to neutralise remaining circulating heparin

3.68   The prothrombin time (PT)

❑   A   measures the activity of the extrinsic coagulation pathway
❑   B   is not usually prolonged in liver disease
❑   C   is prolonged in haemophilia A
❑   D   can be expressed as the INR when monitoring warfarin dosage
❑   E   is prolonged in vitamin K malabsorption

3.69   The following increase the risk of perioperative venous thrombosis

❑   A   sickle cell disease
❑   B   adenocarcinoma of the ovary
❑   C   antithrombin III deficiency
❑   D   increased age
❑   E   ulcerative colitis

3.70   Warfarin

❏ A   impairs the recycling of vitamin K
❏ B   inhibits the synthesis of fibrinogen
❏ C   is best monitored by the activated partial thromboplastin time (APTT)
❏ D   does not affect the bioavailability of antibiotics
❏ E   requires 24 hours to become effective

3.71   Low-molecular-weight heparins (LMWHs)

❏ A   have a mean molecular weight of 15 kDa
❏ B   have a longer half-life than unfractionated heparins
❏ C   act predominantly on factor Xa
❏ D   have a low bioavailability after subcutaneous injection
❏ E   are predominantly eliminated by the kidney

3.72   von Willebrand's disease

❏ A   is a sex-linked disorder
❏ B   is the commonest inherited bleeding disorder in surgical practice
❏ C   is associated with haemarthroses
❏ D   manifests as a prolonged activated partial thromboplastin time (APTT) and bleeding time
❏ E   affected individuals may benefit from preoperative desmopressin

3.73   In the investigation of bleeding disorders

❏ A   bleeding time may be prolonged in patients receiving aspirin
❏ B   fibrinogen concentration is increased in sepsis
❏ C   bleeding time correlates well with the severity of surgical bleeding
❏ D   fibrinogen levels increase in disseminated intravascular coagulation (DIC)
❏ E   thrombin time (TT) is reduced in patients receiving heparin therapy

3.74   The haematological consequences of splenectomy include

❑   A   a thrombocytosis peaking between 3 and 4 months
❑   B   increased circulating Howell–Jolly bodies
❑   C   a reduction in circulating sideroblasts
❑   D   a leucocytosis occurring within hours after the operation
❑   E   reduced platelet adhesiveness

3.75   Acute haemolytic transfusion reactions

❑   A   are most severe if group O cells are transfused into a group A
           recipient
❑   B   may present with loin pain
❑   C   are usually due to ABO typing errors
❑   D   may cause haemoglobinuria
❑   E   are clinically similar to the effects of bacterially contaminated
           blood

3.76   Fat embolism

❑   A   is associated with a petechial rash
❑   B   can be caused by closed fractures
❑   C   is associated with osteoporosis
❑   D   is a complication of long bone fractures
❑   E   produces fat in the sputum
❑   F   typically infarcts in the inferior mesenteric artery
❑   G   may be treatable with steroids

**3.77   The catabolic phase of the metabolic response to trauma is
           characterised by**

❑   A   decreased urine output
❑   B   increased sodium output
❑   C   gluconeogenesis
❑   D   negative nitrogen balance
❑   E   thrombocytosis

3.78   Haemorrhagic shock

❏   A   increases catecholamine secretion by the adrenal cortex
❏   B   causes the oxygen–haemoglobin dissociation curve to shift to
           the left
❏   C   stimulates aortic baroreceptors
❏   D   produces a decrease in ventilation–perfusion mismatch
❏   E   causes an increase in tidal ventilation
❏   F   causes a decrease in atrial pressure and subsequent reduction in
           antidiuretic hormone (ADH) secretion

3.79   Fractures of the frontobasal skull can cause

❏   A   anosmia
❏   B   visual field defects
❏   C   rhinorrhoea
❏   D   retroauricular ecchymoses
❏   E   periorbital ecchymosis

3.80   Extradural haematoma

❏   A   is usually associated with a fracture
❏   B   is usually the result of damage to the anterior branch of the
           middle meningeal artery
❏   C   is typically biconvex on a CT scan
❏   D   is often limited by suture lines
❏   E   is frequently the result of a contre-coup injury

3.81   Tracheostomy

❏   A   may be complicated by tracheal stenosis
❏   B   has to be formally closed after use
❏   C   is a recognised cause of hypothyroidism
❏   D   is best placed at the first tracheal cartilage
❏   E   helps the cough reflex

3.82   Chronic subdural haematoma may cause

❏   A   anosmia
❏   B   rhinorrhoea
❏   C   air in the cranial cavity
❏   D   meningitis
❏   E   gait disturbance
❏   F   seizures

3.83   Features of the crush syndrome include

❏   A   hyperkalaemia
❏   B   oliguria
❏   C   haemoglobinuria
❏   D   methaemoglobinaemia
❏   E   haemoconcentration

3.84   Tachycardia in response to haemorrhage may be absent in the following

❏   A   hypothermia
❏   B   infants
❏   C   a patient with a pacemaker
❏   D   after administration of high-flow oxygen
❏   E   patients on β-blockers

3.85   The early response to trauma (ebb phase) includes

❏   A   an increase in metabolic rate
❏   B   an increase in body temperature
❏   C   an increase in catecholamine levels
❏   D   decreased lactate levels
❏   E   increased glucose levels

3.86   Following trauma, there is

❏   A   increased muscle glycogen breakdown
❏   B   increased insulin secretion
❏   C   an elevation of blood glucose
❏   D   reduced excretion of excess water in the first 48 hours
❏   E   sodium conservation in the first 48 hours

3.87   Recognised features of cardiac tamponade include

❏   A   a 'globular' cardiac outline on chest X-ray (CXR)
❏   B   prominent heart sounds
❏   C   collapsed neck veins
❏   D   pulsus paradoxus
❏   E   hypertension
❏   F   Charcot's triad
❏   G   a possibly normal central venous pressure (CVP)

3.88   The following are typical features of an acute extradural haematoma on CT scan

❏   A   crescent-shaped haematoma
❏   B   haematoma crossing the suture line
❏   C   haematoma crossing the midline
❏   D   associated skull fracture
❏   E   decreased attenuation of the haematoma

3.89   Gastrointestinal consequences of major burns include

❏   A   splanchnic vasodilatation
❏   B   acute gastric dilatation
❏   C   Cushing's ulcers
❏   D   paralytic ileus
❏   E   terminal ileal lymphoid hyperplasia

3.90   Tissue hypoxia secondary to chest trauma may result from

❏   A   pulmonary ventilation–perfusion mismatch
❏   B   hypocarbia
❏   C   hypovolaemia
❏   D   changes in intrathoracic pressure relationships
❏   E   alveolar hypersensitivity

3.91   The following are complications of major burns

❏   A   myoglobinuria
❏   B   hypoglycaemia
❏   C   hyponatraemia
❏   D   sepsis
❏   E   acute appendicitis

3.92   Respiratory insufficiency should be considered with

❏   A PaO_2 of 15 kPa on 40% O_2
❏   B $PaCO_2$ of 5 kPa on 40% O_2
❏   C   the inability to clear secretions
❏   D   a patient with confusion, agitation or drowsiness
❏   E   poor analgesia following abdominal surgery

3.93   Nitrogen balance is positive

❏   A   during the first 3 days following major surgery
❏   B   in sepsis
❏   C   during growth
❏   D   while ACTH levels are high
❏   E   immediately following exercise
❏   F   following bone fractures

3.94   Gas embolus is recognised in

❏   A   hydrogen peroxide wound irrigation
❏   B   criminal abortion
❏   C   varicose vein surgery
❏   D   central line insertion
❏   E   *Clostridium perfringens* infection

3.95   The risk of postoperative renal failure is increased in patients with

❏   A   preoperative sepsis
❏   B   preoperative jaundice
❏   C   preoperative hypertension
❏   D   benign prostatic hypertrophy

3.96   Acute respiratory distress syndrome (ARDS)

❏   A   frequently causes no chest X-ray (CXR) changes
❏   B   produces hyaline fibrosis
❏   C   leads to increased alveolar permeability
❏   D   may occur secondary to septicaemia
❏   E   is commonly managed in a general ward setting

3.97   The following are increased in acute renal failure (ARF)

❑   A   respiratory rate
❑   B   blood pH
❑   C   potassium
❑   D   arterial P_{CO_2}
❑   E   plasma bicarbonate

3.98   Nitric oxide

❑   A   is increased in endotoxic shock
❑   B   causes vasodilatation of smooth muscle
❑   C   is synthesised from inhaled nitrogen
❑   D   causes platelet aggregation
❑   E   is produced from protein metabolism in sepsis

3.99   In acute renal failure

❑   A   fluid resuscitation is rarely required
❑   B   acute cortical necrosis heralds a poor prognosis
❑   C   systemic infection characteristically complicates the illness
❑   D   pain control with non-steroidal anti-inflammatory drugs
            (NSAIDs) should be stopped
❑   E   dialysis should be commenced early

3.100   Complications of an ascending aortic dissection include

❑   A   mitral valve rupture
❑   B   aortic regurgitation
❑   C   cardiac tamponade
❑   D   acute myocardial infarction
❑   E   pulmonary embolus
❑   F   haemothorax

3.101   Causes of ARDS (acute respiratory distress syndrome) include

❑   A   sepsis
❑   B   fat embolism
❑   C   acute pancreatitis
❑   D   acute renal failure
❑   E   burns

3.102 Tracheostomy

❑ A is uncomplicated by thyroid disease
❑ B may be needed for bronchial toilet
❑ C is straightforward in people with a short neck
❑ D will increase the anatomical dead space
❑ E increases the ventilation–perfusion mismatch

3.103 Hazards of artificial ventilation include

❑ A basal atelectasis
❑ B surgical emphysema
❑ C hypotension
❑ D cerebral oedema
❑ E acute gastric dilatation

3.104 Well-recognised causes of hypertension in the postoperative period are

❑ A urinary retention
❑ B pain
❑ C isoflurane
❑ D epidural analgesia
❑ E acute tubular necrosis
❑ F sepsis

3.105 Hypokalaemia

❑ A produces peaked T waves on the ECG
❑ B causes the heart to arrest in diastole
❑ C is seen in metabolic acidosis
❑ D may occur following extensive muscle trauma
❑ E may be seen in pancreatic fistulae
❑ F may be seen in pyloric stenosis

3.106 The following suggest that respiratory failure is chronic rather than acute

❑ A plasma bicarbonate of 39 mmol/l
❑ B PaO_2 of 9 kPa
❑ C PaO_2 of 7 kPa
❑ D arterial pH of 7.2
❑ E the presence of a hypoxic respiratory drive

3.107   Acute renal failure (ARF)

❑   A   is drug-induced in 75% of cases
❑   B   occurs in approximately 30% of critically ill patients
❑   C   may produce little histological change
❑   D   is usually the result of damage to the proximal tubule
❑   E   carries an overall mortality rate of 10%

3.108   Changes in cellular metabolism associated with shock include

❑   A   accumulation of lactic acid
❑   B   increased adenosine triphosphate (ATP) production
❑   C   passage of sodium into cells
❑   D   passage of potassium into cells
❑   E   lysosomal fragmentation
❑   F   increased ketone production

3.109   The management of severe anaphylactic shock may include

❑   A   airway maintenance and oxygen
❑   B   intravenous fluids
❑   C   intra-arterial adrenaline (epinephrine)
❑   D   nebulised bronchoconstrictors
❑   E   β-blockers

3.110   Features of adult respiratory distress syndrome (ARDS) include

❑   A   interstitial and alveolar oedema
❑   B   granulomas
❑   C   hyaline membrane formation
❑   D   glandular hyperplasia
❑   E   interstitial fibrosis

3.111   Perioperative myocardial infarction (MI)

❑   A   most commonly occurs on day 1 postoperatively
❑   B   is more common in patients with a previous infarction
❑   C   is unaffected by the degree of anaesthetic monitoring
❑   D   has a mortality of 50–70%
❑   E   is rare in patients with no previous history of coronary heart disease

3.112   The following tumours and related markers have been correctly paired

- ❏ A   teratoma and α-fetoprotein
- ❏ B   parathyroid tumours and calcitonin
- ❏ C   choriocarcinoma and β-hCG
- ❏ D   serous ovarian cancer and CA-125
- ❏ E   prostate carcinoma and alkaline phosphatase
- ❏ F   cervical cancer and squamous-cell carcinoma antigen

3.113   The following are suggestive of a good prognosis in malignant melanoma

- ❏ A   male sex
- ❏ B   low Breslow thickness
- ❏ C   the presence of ulceration
- ❏ D   older age
- ❏ E   mucosal primary site
- ❏ F   truncal primary site
- ❏ G   white ethnicity

3.114   In devising a suitable screening test for malignant cancer, the

- ❏ A   test should have high specificity
- ❏ B   test should have high sensitivity
- ❏ C   tumour should be of anaplastic type
- ❏ D   tumour should have a short latent phase
- ❏ E   test should be well accepted by the population
- ❏ F   natural history of the disease should be adequately understood

3.115   The following are malignant

- ❏ A   mucosal hamartoma
- ❏ B   sarcoma
- ❏ C   melanoma
- ❏ D   adenoma
- ❏ E   Krukenberg tumour
- ❏ F   Zollinger–Ellison syndrome
- ❏ G   Barrett's oesophagus

3.116   Aggressiveness of a malignant melanoma is suggested by

❑   A   lymphadenopathy
❑   B   bleeding
❑   C   satellite lesions
❑   D   flat lesions
❑   E   amelanotic lesions

3.117   Regarding malignancy

❑   A   this is the second highest cause of mortality in the UK
❑   B   testicular tumours usually spread to inguinal lymph nodes
❑   C   prostatic carcinoma spreads to the vertebrae, bypassing the lungs
❑   D   prostatic tumours are most commonly adenocarcinomas
❑   E   osteosarcoma spreads to the lungs via the thoracic duct

3.118   Beta-naphthylamine is a known cause of

❑   A   small-cell carcinoma of the lung
❑   B   bladder cancer
❑   C   breast cancer
❑   D   adenocarcinoma of the stomach
❑   E   chemical pneumonitis
❑   F   lymphoma

3.119   Staging of malignant tumours

❑   A   helps to establish prognosis
❑   B   includes details of locoregional and distant sites
❑   C   can be made solely on the basis of a histological specimen
❑   D   may be altered by response to irradiation treatment
❑   E   takes into account the local anatomy for individual primary tumour sites

3.120   The following have malignant potential

❑   A   Bowen's disease
❑   B   solar keratosis
❑   C   keratoacanthoma
❑   D   Spitz naevus
❑   E   molluscum contagiosum
❑   F   basal-cell papilloma

3.121 Regarding oncogenes

❏ A they are normal components of cellular molecular physiology
❏ B they code for proteins involved in cell division
❏ C those such as the v-*erbB2* product are overexpressed in colon cancer
❏ D those such as mutated K-*ras* are present in up to 60% of colorectal cancers
❏ E they are expressed during embryogenesis

3.122 Tumour suppressor genes include

❏ A v-*erbB2*
❏ B K-*ras*
❏ C c-*myc*
❏ D retinoblastoma gene (*RB1*)
❏ E *TP53*
❏ F *BRCA1*

3.123 Alpha-fetoprotein levels can be raised in

❏ A nephroblastoma
❏ B hepatocellular carcinoma
❏ C colonic carcinoma
❏ D biliary tumours
❏ E congenital adrenal hyperplasia
❏ F pure seminoma of the testicle
❏ G pregnancy

3.124 The following have a significant metastatic potential

❏ A colonic adenoma
❏ B cholangiocarcinoma
❏ C lipoma
❏ D chondroma
❏ E adenocarcinoma
❏ F fibroadenoma
❏ G basal-cell carcinoma

3.125 Bronchial carcinoma

❑ A when associated with syndrome of inappropriate secretion of antidiuretic hormone (SIADH) suggests irresectability
❑ B can be cured at resection if the mediastinal lymph nodes are also removed
❑ C is associated with *TP53* mutations in 70% cases
❑ D of the small-cell type is relatively radioresistant
❑ E can cause hypokalaemia
❑ F can cause hyponatraemia

3.126 Radiotherapy can be the sole primary treatment for

❑ A adenocarcinoma of oesophagus
❑ B gastric carcinoma
❑ C vocal fold (T1) tumour
❑ D rectal carcinoma
❑ E cystosarcoma phylloides breast tumour
❑ F anal cancer

3.127 The following are premalignant conditions

❑ A familial adenomatous polyposis
❑ B Paget's disease of the nipple
❑ C acanthosis nigricans
❑ D keratoacanthoma
❑ E solar keratosis

3.128 The National Breast Screening Programme

❑ A has led to a major increase in benign breast biopsies
❑ B determines that an interval cancer is one that is detected between screening mammograms
❑ C screens women every 5 years
❑ D is carried out on all women aged between 45 and 65 years of age
❑ E has increased the proportion of T0 disease
❑ F has shown that a quarter of cancers detected are not palpable on physical examination

3.129 Screening

- ❏ A prevents femoral neck fractures
- ❏ B prevents death from cervical cancer
- ❏ C reduces lung cancer mortality
- ❏ D prevents death from medullary carcinoma of the thyroid
- ❏ E prevents death from ovarian cancer

3.130 Malignant tumours may be distinguishable from benign tumours by the presence of

- ❏ A a capsule
- ❏ B a higher mitotic rate
- ❏ C metastasis
- ❏ D oncogene activation
- ❏ E loss of tumour-cell cohesion

3.131 Alkylating agents

- ❏ A can cause myelosuppression
- ❏ B can be antibiotics
- ❏ C include cyclophosphamide
- ❏ D prevent spindle formation
- ❏ E do not cause hair loss

3.132 Neuroblastomas may arise from the

- ❏ A anterior root of the spinal cord
- ❏ B posterior root of the spinal cord
- ❏ C sympathetic chain
- ❏ D adrenal medulla
- ❏ E peripheral nerves

3.133 Serum carcinoembryonic antigen (CEA)

- ❏ A may be useful in the detection of colorectal cancer
- ❏ B is a glycoprotein
- ❏ C is raised in 90% of cases of colorectal cancer
- ❏ D has a mean half-life of 100 days
- ❏ E is elevated in some smokers

3.134 Common carcinogens and their associated malignancies include

❏ A ultraviolet radiation and basal-cell carcinoma
❏ B β-naphthylamine and gastric cancer
❏ C asbestos and mesothelioma
❏ D benzene and colonic cancer
❏ E arsenic and lung cancer

3.135 Cancer registries

❏ A would benefit from an increased hospital postmortem rate
❏ B are only useful for retrospective studies
❏ C are most useful at a local level
❏ D can monitor 5-year survival rates
❏ E have no value in cancer screening

3.136 Hamartomas

❏ A may be present at birth
❏ B arise at the vermilion border of the lip in Peutz–Jeghers syndrome
❏ C are mass lesions
❏ D contain a variety of normal tissue components
❏ E grow autonomously
❏ F grow rapidly in size

3.137 Adenomas

❏ A are typically encapsulated
❏ B can arise in transitional epithelial cells
❏ C typically invade the basement membrane
❏ D are typically annular lesions
❏ E do not contain dysplastic cells

3.138 Oncogenes

❏ A code for proteins involved in cellular regulatory processes
❏ B in some cases encode for growth factors
❏ C must be mutated for carcinogenesis to occur
❏ D exhibit a high degree of evolutionary variability
❏ E may be transmitted by viruses

3.139 **The ability of neoplastic cells to metastasise depends on**

❏ A   tumour angiogenesis
❏ B   decreased cellular cohesion
❏ C   protease secretion
❏ D   reduced cellular adherence to the basement membrane
❏ E   increased production of E-cadherins

3.140 **In the cell cycle**

❏ A   DNA synthesis occurs during the M phase
❏ B   the cell is metabolically inactive in G1 phase
❏ C   the M phase leads to the production of two haploid cells
❏ D   changes in regulatory mechanisms may cause neoplastic transformation
❏ E   the tissue growth rate depends on the length of the S phase

3.141 **Chemotherapy toxicity**

❏ A   is reduced by combination with other chemotherapeutic agents
❏ B   may be increased in hepatic impairment
❏ C   may be treated by serotonin antagonists
❏ D   may present with epistaxis
❏ E   is associated with permanent hair loss
❏ F   is reduced with a higher creatinine clearance

3.142 **Early complications of radiotherapy include**

❏ A   infertility
❏ B   hypothyroidism
❏ C   bone marrow failure
❏ D   mouth ulcers
❏ E   hair loss
❏ F   diarrhoea
❏ G   osteitis

3.143   Known causes of gynaecomastia include

❑ A   bromocriptine
❑ B   cimetidine
❑ C   oral corticosteroids
❑ D   parathyroid gland tumours
❑ E   liver cirrhosis
❑ F   testicular teratomas
❑ G   adrenal gland tumours

3.144   The following are considered to be premalignant conditions

❑ A   Barrett's oesophagus
❑ B   Paget's disease of the breast
❑ C   Peutz–Jeghers syndrome
❑ D   balanitis xerotica obliterans (BXO)
❑ E   familial adenomatous polyposis

3.145   Interpretation of the results of screening programmes for cancer must allow for

❑ A   selection bias
❑ B   calculation bias
❑ C   detection bias
❑ D   length bias
❑ E   lead-time bias

3.146   Oesophageal pathologies that may predispose to oesophageal carcinoma include

❑ A   oesophageal webs
❑ B   pharyngeal pouches
❑ C   corrosive oesophagitis
❑ D   achalasia
❑ E   oesophageal varices
❑ F   hiatus hernia

3.147   The following tumours are related to smoking

- ❏ A   squamous-cell carcinoma of the cervix
- ❏ B   acute myeloid leukaemia
- ❏ C   transitional-cell carcinoma of the bladder
- ❏ D   non-Hodgkin's lymphoma
- ❏ E   carcinoma of the larynx

3.148   Cases that should be referred to the coroner include

- ❏ A   violent death
- ❏ B   death from AIDS
- ❏ C   death from unknown causes
- ❏ D   death from a notifiable disease
- ❏ E   death from anaesthetic
- ❏ F   death from self-neglect
- ❏ G   death while recovering from an anaesthetic
- ❏ H   death related to industrial or occupational disease in former employment

3.149   Informed consent should include discussion about

- ❏ A   per rectal analgesia use
- ❏ B   exact identity of the surgeon
- ❏ C   alternative options
- ❏ D   possible failure
- ❏ E   explanation of the risk of anaesthetic

3.150   Disseminated intravascular coagulation (DIC)

- ❏ A   is confirmed by elevated fibrinogen degradation products
- ❏ B   produces a characteristic raised platelet count
- ❏ C   is best managed with whole blood transfusion
- ❏ D   is associated with increased fibrinolysis
- ❏ E   may present with thrombosis

3.151 Essential components of total parenteral nutrition (TPN) include

❏ A emulsifiers
❏ B nitrogen
❏ C fibrinogen
❏ D carbohydrate
❏ E calcium

3.152 Recognised complications of central venous line insertion include

❏ A arterial air embolism
❏ B haemorrhage
❏ C pneumothorax
❏ D chylothorax
❏ E venous air embolism

3.153 Regarding tumour markers

❏ A they may be useful in monitoring the response to anti-cancer treatment
❏ B they may yield prognostic information
❏ C they play an important role in the management of testicular germ-cell tumours
❏ D they are sufficiently sensitive for screening purposes in the majority of cases
❏ E CA-125 is found in the normal ovary
❏ F Prostate-specific antigen (PSA) is found in the normal prostate

3.154 Malignant tumours can be differentiated from benign tumours on the basis of

❏ A the presence of a capsule
❏ B metastases
❏ C a slow growth rate
❏ D poor differentiation of cells
❏ E cells of differing sizes

3.155 Thrombophlebitis migrans is associated with

- ❑ A carcinoma of pancreas
- ❑ B phlegmasia cerulae dolens
- ❑ C bronchial carcinoma
- ❑ D venous insufficiency
- ❑ E diabetes
- ❑ F Lyme disease

3.156 Concerning viral hepatitis

- ❑ A hepatitis A is an RNA virus
- ❑ B hepatitis B is an RNA virus
- ❑ C hepatitis A has an incubation period of 2–5 days
- ❑ D hepatitis A rarely causes fulminant hepatitis
- ❑ E hepatitis A may give rise to a carrier state

3.157 Infectious causes of abdominal pain in HIV-infected individuals include

- ❑ A *Cryptosporidium*
- ❑ B cytomegalovirus
- ❑ C *Clostridium perfringens*
- ❑ D Kaposi's sarcoma
- ❑ E *Mycobacterium tuberculosis*

3.158 *Streptococcus pyogenes*

- ❑ A produces an erythrogenic toxin
- ❑ B is α-haemolytic
- ❑ C belongs to Lancefield group A
- ❑ D is found in clusters
- ❑ E is sensitive to tetracycline
- ❑ F is associated with glomerulonephritis

3.159 Correct pairings of the organ and predominant commensal bacterial flora include

- ❑ A skin and coliforms
- ❑ B lower respiratory tract and streptococci
- ❑ C oropharynx and streptococci
- ❑ D large bowel and *Bacteroides fragilis*
- ❑ E vagina and lactobacillus

3.160   Phagocytosis involves

❏   A   release of lysosomal products
❏   B   lymphocyte activation
❏   C   interleukin release
❏   D   hydrogen peroxide
❏   E   elastase release

3.161   Intravascular haemolysis

❏   A   seldom occurs after ABO-mismatched blood transfusion
❏   B   may occur after burns
❏   C   is common in autoimmune haemolytic anaemia
❏   D   may occur in disseminated intravascular coagulation (DIC)
❏   E   may occur after mitral valve replacement

3.162   Characteristic features of haemorrhagic shock include

❏   A   coma
❏   B   reduced urine output
❏   C   decreased peripheral vascular resistance
❏   D   bradycardia
❏   E   hypotension

3.163   Acute circulatory failure with a high central venous pressure (CVP) and a low blood pressure can be seen in

❏   A   haemorrhage
❏   B   congestive cardiac failure
❏   C   septicaemia
❏   D   tension pneumothorax
❏   E   venous air embolism
❏   F   pulmonary embolism
❏   G   myocardial infarction
❏   H   fast atrial fibrillation

3.164 Acute renal failure (ARF)

❏ A   may lead to elevated plasma calcium and PO_2 levels
❏ B   carries an increased risk of gastrointestinal tract bleeding
❏ C   is usually associated with urinary sodium excretion > 20 mmol/l
❏ D   produces a urine osmolality > 400 mOsm/l
❏ E   if persisting for longer than 4 weeks, patients should undergo a renal biopsy

3.165 The catabolic phase of the metabolic response to injury

❏ A   is accompanied by increased energy expenditure
❏ B   is accompanied by a positive nitrogen balance
❏ C   varies in response to the severity of the trauma
❏ D   is most dramatic following multisystem trauma and extensive burns
❏ E   is prolonged by sepsis

3.166 The following are malignant

❏ A   lymphoma
❏ B   meningioma
❏ C   rhabdomyoma
❏ D   melanoma
❏ E   chondrosarcoma

3.167 Metastatic spread

❏ A   commonly occurs transluminally
❏ B   via the lymphatics is a common feature of basal-cell carcinoma
❏ C   via the lymphatics is a feature of osteosarcoma
❏ D   via the blood is a common feature of prostatic carcinoma
❏ E   to regional lymph nodes usually follows the pattern of venous drainage

3.168   Hypercalcaemia may be associated with

❑   A   carcinoma of the bronchus
❑   B   prolonged immobilisation
❑   C   hypoparathyroidism
❑   D   blood transfusion
❑   E   multiple myeloma
❑   F   renal insufficiency
❑   G   hyperthyroidism

3.169   The following skin lesions have malignant potential

❑   A   squamous cell
❑   B   Merkel cell
❑   C   dermatofibroma
❑   D   Bowen's disease
❑   E   solar keratosis

3.170   Tourniquet

❑   A   may be safely inflated for 60 minutes (constant duration) in the upper limb
❑   B   application does not affect nerve conduction
❑   C   should be released before a wound is sutured
❑   D   pressure should be between arterial and venous pressures
❑   E   is used as part of a Bier's block technique for upper limb anaesthesia

3.171   In the healing of adult bone

❑   A   the stimulation of osteoprogenitor cells by factors such as FGF and PDGF play an important role
❑   B   the histological appearance resembles that in an osteosarcoma
❑   C   internal fixation reduces callus formation
❑   D   a fracture haematoma delays healing by maintaining a degree of separation between the bone-ends
❑   E   callus formation can be seen on an X-ray by 10 days

3.172   Late complications of fractures include

❏   A   infection
❏   B   Volkmann's ischaemic contracture
❏   C   tendon rupture
❏   D   myositis ossificans
❏   E   algodystrophy

3.173   Fracture non-union

❏   A   may occur if the fracture surfaces are interposed by muscle
❏   B   characteristically produces painless movement at the fracture site
❏   C   always requires treatment
❏   D   may be treated by electrical stimulation
❏   E   may require bone grafting if of the atrophic type

3.174   Delayed fracture union

❏   A   is rarely seen in the lower tibia
❏   B   may be caused by an intact fellow bone
❏   C   produces a tender fracture site
❏   D   produces a marked periosteal reaction
❏   E   may be treated by functional bracing

3.175   Paget's disease of bone

❏   A   characteristically affects the cortex
❏   B   can be treated with bisphosphonates
❏   C   causes an elevated alkaline phosphatase
❏   D   is uncommon in patients under 50 years of age
❏   E   is most commonly found in the femur
❏   F   predisposes to fractures
❏   G   can be treated with calcium

3.176   Postoperative osteomyelitis

❏   A   often produces tenderness and pain on movement of the limb
❏   B   may be accurately diagnosed by MRI in the early stages
❏   C   is more likely if there is implant loosening
❏   D   is eliminated by prophylactic antibiotics
❏   E   is usually due to a single bacterial pathogen

3.177 Avascular necrosis is a well-recognised complication of

❏ A a fracture of the proximal pole of the scaphoid
❏ B a supracondylar fracture of the distal humerus
❏ C an intertrochanteric fracture of the femoral neck
❏ D a fracture of the talar neck
❏ E a fracture of the hook of the hamate

3.178 Acute osteomyelitis

❏ A is usually caused by *Streptococcus pyogenes*
❏ B may occur from a skin abrasion
❏ C usually begins in the metaphysis
❏ D is more common in the vertebrae in adults
❏ E has normal X-ray appearances during the first 10 days

3.179 The following are causes of leg lymphoedema

❏ A familial predisposition
❏ B angio-oedema
❏ C *Wuchereria bancrofti* infection
❏ D radiotherapy
❏ E Klippel–Trenaunay syndrome

3.180 In vascular thrombosis

❏ A 'coralline clot' is also known as 'red thrombus'
❏ B 'propagative clot' is also known as 'white thrombus'
❏ C 'red thrombus' has little adherence to the vessel wall and is
         particularly likely to break up and form emboli
❏ D anticoagulants have little effect on platelet aggregation
❏ E thrombophlebitis is associated with a clinical inflammatory
         reaction

3.181 Branchial cysts

❏ A pass between the inferior and middle constrictors
❏ B contain cholesterol crystals
❏ C frequently become infected
❏ D may present in childhood

3.182   Concerning parotid adenoma

❑   A   it is the commonest salivary neoplasm
❑   B   it is found in the deep and superficial parts of the gland
❑   C   it characteristically produces a facial nerve palsy
❑   D   it is more common in men
❑   E   Frey's syndrome is a complication of parotid surgery

3.183   Parotid gland tumours

❑   A   account for approximately 80% of all salivary gland tumours
❑   B   are most commonly benign
❑   C   are always slow-growing
❑   D   can present with otalgia
❑   E   can be core biopsied safely under MRI guidance

3.184   Causes of hypercalcaemia include

❑   A   Addison's disease
❑   B   renal failure
❑   C   diabetes mellitus
❑   D   sarcoidosis
❑   E   thyrotoxicosis

3.185   Long-term effects of gastrectomy include

❑   A   low serum iron
❑   B   renal calculi
❑   C   osteomalacia
❑   D   vitamin B_{12} deficiency
❑   E   vitamin C deficiency

3.186   Squamous-cell carcinoma of the anal canal

❑   A   may spread to pelvic lymph nodes
❑   B   is associated with human papillomavirus infection
❑   C   characteristically presents with faecal incontinence
❑   D   is relatively radioresistant
❑   E   is related to increased dietary fat intake

3.187   Features more likely to be associated with Crohn's disease than ulcerative colitis (UC) include

❏   A   stricture formation
❏   B   obstruction
❏   C   fistula formation
❏   D   cancer
❏   E   perianal involvement

3.188   Horseshoe kidney

❏   A   is more common in women
❏   B   usually has a standard blood supply
❏   C   is more prone to infection
❏   D   is more prone to trauma
❏   E   may complicate aortic aneurysm repair

3.189   Neuropathic bladder dysfunction is associated with

❏   A   spina bifida
❏   B   diabetes mellitus
❏   C   abdominal hysterectomy
❏   D   anterior resection
❏   E   vesicoureteric reflux

3.190   The following stones form in acidic urine

❏   A   cysteine
❏   B   staghorn calculi
❏   C   urate calculi
❏   D   calcium phosphate
❏   E   struvite calculi

3.191   Osteosarcoma

❏   A   affects the epiphysis of the long bones
❏   B   usually presents between the ages of 30 and 50 years
❏   C   is a recognised complication of Paget's disease
❏   D   produces increased bone formation
❏   E   complicates osteochondroma

3.192   Conduction deafness is caused by

- ❏   A   Paget's disease of the bone
- ❏   B   an acoustic neuroma
- ❏   C   otosclerosis
- ❏   D   a fracture through the petrous temporal bone
- ❏   E   otitis media

3.193   Meckel's diverticulum

- ❏   A   is invariably found in the jejunum
- ❏   B   is a recognised cause of malabsorption
- ❏   C   should not be removed if found incidentally
- ❏   D   may present with rectal bleeding
- ❏   E   may lead to macrocytic anaemia
- ❏   F   is found in over 20% of the general population
- ❏   G   is a true diverticulum
- ❏   H   is associated with a patent urachus

3.194   Amyloidosis is seen in

- ❏   A   papillary carcinoma of thyroid
- ❏   B   acute pancreatitis
- ❏   C   multiple myeloma
- ❏   D   dialysis patients
- ❏   E   rheumatoid arthritis

3.195   Postsplenectomy sepsis

- ❏   A   is more common in adults than in children
- ❏   B   may be due to *Streptococcus pneumoniae*
- ❏   C   may be due to *Haemophilus influenzae*
- ❏   D   may be prevented by daily penicillin
- ❏   E   may be due to *Neisseria meningitidis*

3.196   Causes of massive splenomegaly include

- ❏   A   Chagas' disease
- ❏   B   malaria
- ❏   C   chronic hepatitis C
- ❏   D   chronic myeloid leukaemia
- ❏   E   myelofibrosis

3.197 Keloid scars

❑ A are treated by triamcinolone injections
❑ B may occur on mucosal surfaces
❑ C should be treated by surgery
❑ D rarely occur in the mid-sternal region
❑ E should be treated by radiotherapy
❑ F are reduced along Langer's lines
❑ G may give rise to contractures across joint lines

3.198 The following tumours are associated with the given risk factors

❑ A scrotal carcinoma and chimney sweeps
❑ B bladder cancer and dye workers
❑ C renal transitional-cell carcinoma and phenacetin abuse
❑ D penile cancer and circumcision
❑ E prostate cancer and vasectomy

3.199 Secondary haemorrhage

❑ A occurs within 24 hours
❑ B may be massive
❑ C usually requires a blood transfusion
❑ D may be associated with a deep infection
❑ E is the result of anticoagulation

3.200 A fall in serum calcium levels causes

❑ A reduced osteoclastic activity
❑ B increased vitamin D production
❑ C increased bone resorption
❑ D reduced parathyroid hormone (PTH) secretion
❑ E renal tubule impermeability to calcium

3.201 Acute respiratory distress syndrome (ARDS)

❑ A is characterised by decreased lung compliance
❑ B is caused due to collapse of the alveoli
❑ C has an increased PaO_2 (in mmHg) to FIO_2 ratio
❑ D can lead to pulmonary fibrosis
❑ E has > 50% mortality is established cases

ANSWERS

SECTION 1: ANATOMY – ANSWERS

1.1 CDE
Children have a relatively larger head which tends to flex the head on the neck, making airway obstruction more likely. The relatively larger tongue tends to flop back and obstruct the airway in the obtunded child which means that there is less room in the mouth when intubation is being carried out. The larynx is positioned more cephalic (glottis at C3 in infants compared with C6 in adults) and the angle of the jaw is larger in children (140° in infants, 120° in adults), both of which make intubation more difficult. In addition, the trachea is shorter and the cricoid ring is the narrowest part of the airway (compared with the glottis in the adult).

1.2 AD
Below the L1 vertebra (transpyloric plane), the anterior and posterior nerve roots pass almost vertically downwards through the subarachnoid space and form the cauda equina. This consists only of anterior and posterior nerve roots. The subcostal plane lies at L3. A positive Babinski sign represents an upper motor neurone defect.

1.3 CE
Damage to the long thoracic nerve causes winging of the scapula owing to weakness of the serratus anterior. Spinal accessory nerve damage will cause weakness in shrugging the shoulders. The axillary nerve contains fibres of C5 and C6 to supply predominantly the deltoid muscle. It conveys some sensory fibres to the lateral aspect of the forearm. The radial nerve supplies the extensor carpi radialis and ulnaris, plus extensor digitorum, so its injury results in wrist drop. Froment's (pincer) sign is associated with an ulnar nerve injury, where the adductor pollicis is weak and so the flexor pollicis longus accommodates. When a sheet of paper is placed between the thumb and index finger of a patient with a weak adductor pollicis, he/she will flex the thumb at the interphalangeal joint to grip the sheet. Sciatic nerve injuries result in foot drop, so the high-stepping gait.

1.4 ACD
Cervical cord injury is characterised by flaccid areflexia, diaphragmatic breathing and the ability to flex but not extend the elbow. Priapism is an uncommon but characteristic sign. Full immobilisation of the neck is required at all times.

1.5   AC

Cerebrospinal fluid is predominantly produced by the choroid plexuses in the ventricles, which are connected via the foramen of Monro. CSF is produced at a rate of 0.3–0.5 ml/h. The arachnoid granulations (villi) are involved in the reabsorption of CSF into the venous sinuses and so into the systemic circulation.

1.6   BD

Cerebral perfusion pressure is calculated by the mean arterial blood pressure minus the intracranial pressure. It is tightly regulated so that perfusion pressure, and hence cerebral blood flow, fluctuates very little despite many postural changes. The autoregulatory stimuli are Po_2 and pH (Pco_2 exerts its effect via dissociation into bicarbonate and hydrogen ions and hence a fall in pH). Mannitol is used to reduce intracranial oedema, and hence intracranial pressure, in cases of head injury. This has the effect of increasing cerebral blood flow, but it has no effect in normal subjects.

1.7   E

A collapsed L5–S1 disc presses on the S1 spinal nerve (the L5 nerve passes above the prolapsed disc in the intervertebral foramen and so escapes damage). At the level of prolapse, the spinal canal contains the cauda equina and not cord *per se*. The S1 dermatome lies over the lateral malleolus. Exaggerated reflexes are diagnostic of an upper motor neurone lesion. The S2 dermatome occupies the posterior aspect of the calf.

1.8   AD

The femoral nerve supplies the quadratus femoris muscle, the contracting fibres of which elicit the knee jerk. The nerve supplies the L2–L4 dermatomes over the anterior skin of the thigh. The genitofemoral nerve mediates the cremasteric reflex. The saphenous nerve (L4), a branch of the femoral nerve, innervates the skin over the medial malleolus. The lateral cutaneous nerve of the thigh, and the genitofemoral nerve, both branches of the lumbar plexus, also supply the L2 dermatome.

1.9   BCDE
The odontoid peg is the ascension of the atlas fused to the ascension of the axis. The peg has an articular facet at its front and forms part of a joint with the anterior arch of the atlas. It is a non-weight-bearing joint. The alar ligaments, together with the apical ligaments, are attached from the sloping upper edge of the odontoid peg to the margins of the foramen magnum. The inner ligaments limit rotation of the head and are very strong. The weak apical ligament lies in front of the upper longitudinal bone of the cruciform ligament, and joins the apex of the deltoid peg to the anterior margin of the foramen magnum. It is the fibrous remnant of the notochord.

1.10   DE
Abduction of the thumb is weakened, but not lost, after paralysis of the abductor pollicis longus muscle (radial nerve), because the abductor pollicis brevis muscle remains functional (median nerve). Extension of the forearm is unaffected, since branches to the triceps muscle leave the radial nerve before it enters the spiral groove. Despite paralysis of the supinator muscle, supination is unaffected because the biceps muscle remains functional (musculocutaneous nerve). Loss of sensation over the first dorsal web and of the brachioradialis tendon reflex (mainly C6 through a branch coming off the radial nerve after leaving the spiral groove) are features of radial nerve damage at this site.

1.11   BCD
The branches of the posterior cord are the upper and lower subscapular, thoracodorsal and axillary nerves. It terminates as the radial nerve. Through the axillary nerve, the posterior cord supplies the deltoid muscle. The musculocutaneous nerve leaves the lateral cord to supply the coracobrachialis muscle. The suprascapular nerve supplies the infra- and supraspinatous muscles and is derived from the upper trunk.

1.12   C
Signs of S1 nerve root compression include: reduced sensation in the S1 dermatome (sole of the foot); weakness of plantar flexion of the ankle; and absent or reduced ankle jerk.

1.13   BD

Ulnar nerve damage results in sensory loss over the hypothenar eminence, the whole of the little finger and the medial side of the ring finger. There is denervation of the flexor carpi ulnaris muscle, the ulnar half of the flexor digitorum profundus muscle, the muscles of the hypothenar eminence, the two ulnar lumbricals, all the interosseous muscles and the adductor pollicis muscle. So, both flexion of the little finger and abduction of the fingers are lost. Adduction of the wrist is still possible through the action of the extensor carpi ulnaris muscle. Claw hand, a feature of ulnar nerve damage at the wrist, is usually not present with high lesions at the elbow or above, because the distal interphalangeal joints cannot be flexed if the ulnar half of the flexor digitorum profundus muscle is paralysed.

1.14   BCD

In Erb's palsy (traction injury of the upper roots and trunk – C5/6), there is paralysis of the abductors and lateral rotators of the shoulder, the elbow flexors and the supinator muscles. The arm hangs by the side medially rotated, extended at the elbow, and pronated. There is also loss of cutaneous sensation over the lateral aspect of the arm and forearm.

1.15   ABE

The left coronary artery arises from the left posterior aortic sinus behind the pulmonary trunk. After a short course it divides into two main arteries, the circumflex artery and the left anterior descending artery, otherwise known as the anterior interventricular artery: 60% of hearts have the right coronary artery supplying the SA node; in 40% of hearts, the SA nodal artery arises from the left coronary artery. The left coronary artery supplies the vast majority of the left ventricle and left atrium. Part of the right ventricle is supplied by the left coronary artery through a conus branch.

1.16   DE

The scalenus anterior is attached to the scalene tubercle. The scalenus medius is attached to the area behind the posterior groove. The subclavian artery passes anterior to the first thoracic nerve root.

1.17   BCDE
Each half of the diaphragm is supplied by its own phrenic nerve (C3, C4, C5) which is both motor and sensory. The intercostal nerves send some proprioceptive fibres to the periphery of the diaphragm. The oesophageal opening is opposite the T10 vertebra behind the seventh costal cartilage. It lies in the fibres of the left crus, but a sling of fibres from the right crus loops around it. The greater, lesser and least splanchnic nerves pierce each crus.

1.18   BDE
An intercostal drain should be inserted in the fifth intercostal space in the mid-axillary line and so should not penetrate pectoralis major. The visceral pleura overlies the lung and should not be entered, although this may occur inadvertently.

1.19   BDF
The phrenic nerve is sensory and motor to the diaphragm. The main motor root is C5 and injury to the phrenic nerve causes paralysis of the corresponding hemidiaphragm. This leads to paradoxical movement of the diaphragm, rising on inspiration.

1.20   ADE
The vertical dimension of the chest increases on inspiration. The ribs move upwards and outwards. However, the first rib does not move during respiration. The serratus anterior (supplied by the long thoracic nerve) is involved in respiration.

1.21   C
A CT section at this level is at the level of T4. At this level, the arch of the aorta is terminating, the azygos vein enters the superior vena cava (SVC), the left recurrent laryngeal nerve loops round the ligamentum venosum and the bifurcation of the pulmonary trunk can be seen. The thoracic duct crosses the midline at T5.

1.22   BE
Bleeding from the middle meningeal artery following head injury usually leads to an extradural haematoma. This is usually a tear of the anterior branch of the middle meningeal artery, with an underlying linear skull fracture. The characteristic picture is of a head injury with a brief episode of unconsciousness followed by a lucid interval. The patient then develops a progressive hemiparesis, stupor and rapid transtentorial coning with an ipsilateral dilated pupil. This is followed by bilateral fixed dilated pupils, tetraplegia and death.

1.23   ADE

The left lung has two lobes, in contrast to the right, which has three lobes. The left lung has two bronchial openings and ten bronchopulmonary segments. Two pulmonary veins arise from the left lung, one above and one below the oblique fissure. The arterial supply is from the bronchial arteries which arise from the aorta.

1.24   AC

The foramen spinosum transmits the middle meningeal vessels and the meningeal branch of the mandibular nerve. The foramen rotundum contains the maxillary nerve. The foramen ovale transmits the mandibular nerve, lesser petrosal nerve and accessory meningeal artery. The foramen lacerum transmits the internal carotid and greater petrosal nerve, which leaves as a nerve of the pterygoid canal.

1.25   ABCE

The right main bronchus is shorter (approximately 2.5 cm long), wider and runs more vertically than the left main bronchus. The right main bronchus gives off the upper lobe branch (before entering the lung) and passes inferior to the pulmonary artery before entering the hilum of the lung (approximately T5). It is important to remember the azygos vein, which arches over the right main bronchus from the posterior aspect as it passes to the SVC, and the pulmonary artery, which lies inferior and then anterior to it. The left main bronchus is about 5 cm long and, unlike the right, does not give off any branches before entering the hilum of the left lung at the level of T6.

1.26   CE

The recurrent laryngeal nerve supplies all the intrinsic muscles of the larynx except the cricothyroid and is sensory inferior to the vocal folds. In the neck the recurrent laryngeal nerves on both sides follow the same course, ascending in the tracheo-oesophageal groove. As the nerve passes the lateral lobe of the thyroid it is closely related to the inferior thyroid artery. The superior laryngeal nerve supplies the vocal cord mucosa.

1.27   All true
The external jugular vein drains most of the scalp and side of the face. It begins near the angle of the mandible and is formed from the union of retromandibular and postauricular veins, receiving branches from the posterior external and transverse cervical veins. The external jugular vein has no valves, lies anterior to scalenus anterior and pierces the deep fascia of the neck, usually posterior to the clavicular head of the sternocleido-mastoid muscle before draining into the subclavian vein.

1.28   ABE
The left main bronchus passes downwards and outwards below the aortic arch, anterior to the descending aorta and oesophagus. The pulmonary artery loops over it, the vagus nerve lies just posterior, the phrenic nerve in front, and the hemiazygos vein is posterior to the aorta.

1.29   All true
The sinoatrial node artery passes backwards between the right auricle and aorta, and forms a vascular ring around the termination of the superior vena cava. Arteriolar anastomoses between the terminations of the right and left coronary arteries exist, but are too few and small in calibre to compensate significantly in acute coronary artery occlusion.

1.30   ABCD
The right atrium forms the right border of the heart, lies anterior to the left atrium and so the posterior wall is the interatrial septum. The sinoatrial node lies near the opening of the superior vena cava, lateral to the sulcus limitans, and the coronary sinus opens into the atrium above both the opening of the inferior vena cava and the septal cusp of the tricuspid valve.

1.31   BCDE
The left crus is attached to the L1/2 vertebrae, and both crura are pierced by the sympathetic splanchnic nerves. Inferior phrenic arteries (the first branches of the abdominal aorta) supply the diaphragm. Both suprarenal glands lie against the diaphragm retroperitoneally. Both kidneys lie on the lateral arcuate ligaments and so a pneumothorax is a possible complication of nephrectomy.

1.32   BE

The vagus nerve lies just posterior to the right main bronchus and the azygos vein is at first posterior and then arches over the bronchus. The phrenic nerve is anterior to the bronchus. The right recurrent laryngeal nerve hooks around the right subclavian artery superior to the right main bronchus.

1.33   All true

The thyroid gland is supplied by the inferior thyroid artery, a branch of the thyrocervical trunk. The internal thoracic artery supplies: the breast, through anterior intercostal vessels, usually in the second and third intercostal spaces; the rectus abdominis muscle, through the superior epigastric branch; and the diaphragm, through the musculophrenic artery. The vertebral arteries supply the brainstem through the posterior inferior cerebellar arteries.

1.34   ABDE

The phrenic nerve lies anterior and the vagus posterior to the left hilum. The left main bronchus lies inferior and posterior to the pulmonary artery and does not divide before entering the lung. The hilum is separated from the aortic arch and descending thoracic aorta by the vagus nerve.

1.35   CE

The central tendon is pierced by the inferior vena cava and right phrenic nerve (caval opening) at the level of T8 and the sixth costal cartilage. The vagal trunks, oesophagus and left gastric vessels pass through the oesophageal opening in the muscle of the right crus (T10). The greater splanchnic nerves pierce the crura. The aorta, azygos and hemiazygos veins, as well as the thoracic duct, pass posterior to the diaphragm through the aortic aperture.

1.36   BDE

The apex of the arch, which gives attachment to the pretracheal fascia, lies posteroinferior to the left brachiocephalic vein. The lower border of the arch lies in the transthoracic plane and on the left is directly related to the left pulmonary artery (the superior vena cava lies over the right pulmonary artery). The arch is symmetrically covered by the pleura from both sides, which meet in the midline behind the manubriosternal joint.

1.37   ABCD

The autonomic fibres in the phrenic nerve are sympathetic and pass from the superior (C1–C4) and middle (C5/6) sympathetic cervical ganglia as grey rami into the C3–C5 roots of the phrenic nerve, and innervate blood vessels in the diaphragm. The nerve lies on the fibrous pericardium and is sensory to the mediastinal and diaphragmatic pleura, and also to the diaphragmatic peritoneum. The phrenic nerve enters the chest by descending from the medial lower border of the scalenus anterior muscle between the subclavian vein anteriorly and artery posteriorly.

1.38   AC

Impressions on the mediastinal surface of the right lung include the trachea, vagus, superior vena cava, right atrium and subclavian artery. The oesophagus grooves the left lung above the arch of the aorta and below the hilum.

1.39   ABE

The trachea commences at the lower border of the cricoid cartilage, is palpable in the jugular notch, bifurcates in the transthoracic plane and is innervated by the recurrent laryngeal nerves. The left main bronchus bifurcates inside the left lung and is not as vertical as the right main bronchus.

1.40   AC

The breast lies on the pectoralis major, serratus anterior and external oblique muscles. It is a modified apocrine sweat gland. The mammary gland is mainly supplied by the lateral thoracic artery, by branches that curl around the border of pectoralis major. In addition, there is a blood supply from the internal thoracic artery, intercostal and thoracoacromial arteries. The main lymphatic drainage is to the axillary and infraclavicular nodes. The gland contains approximately 15 main ducts that open separately on the summit of the nipple.

1.41   AB

The blood supply to the breast is mainly from the lateral thoracic artery. The internal thoracic artery, perforating intercostal arteries and the pectoral branches of the thoracoacromial artery also contribute. Venous return simply follows the arteries mentioned above. The nipple is a reasonable reliable marker for the T4 dermatome. In the breast, 75% of the lymphatic drainage is via the axillary nodes. The retromammary space overlies the pectoralis major muscle.

1.42   AE

The clavipectoral fascia arises from the clavicle and encloses pectoralis minor before fusing with the floor of the axilla. The thoracodorsal nerve supplies latissimus dorsi. Damage to the long thoracic nerve (serratus anterior) causes a winged scapula. Level I nodes lie lateral to the pectoralis minor, level II behind and level III medial to pectoralis minor. Division of the intercostobrachial nerve (T2) can lead to anaesthesia on the medial aspect of the upper arm.

1.43   ABCD

Small lymphatic vessels from the breast cross the midline to the other breast, and also cross the diaphragm, where they communicate with the whole breast and the lymphatics of the liver. The regional lymph nodes of the breast are found in the axilla and drain mainly the superior and lateral aspects, while those along the internal mammary artery may drain the inferior and medial parts. The subclavian lymph trunk emerges from the apical nodes of the axilla, and on the right drains into the subclavian vein or right jugular trunk. On the left it usually drains into the thoracic duct.

1.44   ACE

The cisterna chyli runs between the aorta and the right crus of the diaphragm, passes through the aortic diaphragm opening and drains into the thoracic duct. The thoracic duct ascends anterior to the posterior intercostal vessels and has several valves. At the thoracic inlet, it lies to the left of the oesophagus and arches forward over the dome of the left pleura, draining into the left brachiocephalic vein. The right bronchomediastinal trunk drains into the right subclavian vein.

1.45   ACE

The phrenic nerve arises from C3, C4 and C5 deep to the scalenus anterior and medius muscles, and runs on scalenus anterior, over the anterior part of the dome of the pleura, to enter the mediastinum posterior to the subclavian vein. Here the right phrenic nerve spirals forward to lie on the SVC, right atrium and inferior vena cava (IVC), and traverses the diaphragm via the caval orifice. The vagus nerve gives off the recurrent laryngeal nerve.

1.46   ACDE
The common peroneal nerve supplies the lateral and anterior muscular compartments of the calf as well as the skin over the anterior aspects of the calf and foot. With foot drop, the patient trips on walking, as the toes catch the ground. Cutaneous innervation of the sole of the foot is through the medial and lateral plantar branches of the tibial nerve. Inversion is weakened because of paralysis of the tibialis anterior muscle. Muscle wasting is a sign of lower motor neurone damage. The peroneus longus tendon is one of the supports of the lateral arch; when this is paralysed, the arch is compromised.

1.47   ABD
The thoracic sympathetic chain lies on the heads of the ribs, anterior to the posterior intercostal vessels, immediately under cover of the pleura, with the splanchnic nerves passing from the chain medially and anteriorly over the vertebral bodies. The thoracic sympathetic chain receives white rami from all the intercostal nerves, and passes into the abdomen under the medial arcuate ligament of the diaphragm.

1.48   ADE
The scalenus anterior inserts on the scalene tubercule. A groove is found on the first rib anterior to the scalene tubercule for the subclavian vein. The subclavian artery runs behind the scalenus anterior muscle. The first rib is related to the lower two roots of the brachial plexus, C8 and T1. The cervicothoracic ganglion, otherwise known as the 'stellate ganglion', lies in front of the neck of the first rib.

1.49   A
The oesophagus is formed at the lower border of the cricoid cartilage. It is crossed anteriorly by the left main bronchus, lies behind the left atrium and passes through the muscular part of the diaphragm to the left of the central tendon, through the muscular sling of the left crus. It is innervated, in part, by the recurrent laryngeal nerve, not the phrenic nerve.

1.50   DE
The clavipectoral fascia is pierced by the cephalic vein and lateral pectoral nerve, overlain by the C4 dermatome (acromial branches of the supraclavicular nerves), and the infraclavicular lymph nodes. The fascia splits to enclose the pectoralis minor and subclavius muscles, and continues beyond as the suspensory ligament of the axilla.

1.51   ACDE

The left brachiocephalic vein drains blood from: the cervical vertebrae via both vertebral veins; the thyroid gland by the inferior thyroid veins; the first left intercostal space via the left superior intercostal veins; and all the anterior intercostal spaces by the anterior intercostal veins draining into the internal thoracic veins. The thoracic duct enters the vein at its commencement behind the left sternoclavicular joint. The bronchial veins drain into the azygos/hemiazygos systems.

1.52   ABDE

The femoral (Scarpa's) triangle is a fascial space in the medial upper thigh. Its sides are formed superiorly by the inguinal ligament, medially by the adductor longus and laterally by the sartorius muscles. The floor is formed by the iliopsoas, pectineus and adductor longus muscles. The triangle contains the femoral vessels and nerve. Within the femoral triangle, the femoral artery divides into its deep and superficial branches; and the femoral vein receives deep femoral and saphenous tributaries.

1.53   ACE

The greater sciatic notch is converted into the greater sciatic foramen by the sacrospinous ligament. This foramen transmits many structures between the gluteal and pelvic regions including superior and inferior gluteal vessels and nerves; sciatic nerve; posterior cutaneous nerve of the thigh; the nerve to obturator internus and quadratus femoris; the pudendal nerve; and the internal pudendal vessels. The lesser sciatic foramen is the space between the sacrospinous and sacrotuberous ligaments. It contains: the pudendal nerve; the nerve and tendon to obturator internus; and the internal pudendal vessels. The pudendal nerve and the internal pudendal vessels exit the pelvis via the greater sciatic foramen and enter the perineum through the lesser sciatic foramen. Similarly, the nerve to the obturator internus leaves the pelvis via the greater sciatic foramen and soon re-enters the pelvis through the lesser sciatic foramen.

1.54   ACD
The femoral sheath is a downward continuation of the abdominal fascia about 2.5 cm below the inguinal ligament. It is believed to allow for femoral vessel movement in the inguinal region during movement of the hip. The mnemonic 'NAVEL' describes some of the key structures in this region (from lateral to medial): femoral nerve, artery, vein, empty space, lymphatics (Cloquet's). Apart from the femoral nerve, that lies most laterally, all the other structures in the mnemonic are encased in the femoral sheath. The mentioned empty space and lymphatic compartments form the 'femoral canal', where femoral hernias may occur. Therefore, the femoral canal is in the most medial portion of the femoral sheath. The femoral ring is the abdominal opening into the femoral canal. At 2–3 cm below the inguinal ligament, the femoral sheath fuses with the adventitia of the femoral vessels. The pubic branch of the inferior epigastric artery replaces the obturator artery in about 30% of cases, and may be at risk in a femoral hernia repair.

1.55   BD
The Trendelenburg test is used to assess stability of the hip. A positive Trendelenburg test is seen with any painful disorder of the hip. It is also present with a dislocated or subluxed hip and in other conditions where the proximal femoral anatomy is abnormal (short femoral neck with high-riding trochanter). Weak abductor muscles will also lead to a positive test. The abductors of the hip include piriformis, gluteus medius and minimis. Pectineus adducts the hip. The other adductors of the hip are gracilis, and adductor longus, brevis and magnus.

1.56   AB
The roof of the popliteal fossa is formed by the fascia lata. Within the apex of the fossa the sciatic nerve divides into common peroneal and tibial branches (but may divide higher), the former lying either against or under the medial edge of the biceps femoris muscle. The deepest structure is the popliteal artery. The sural nerve pierces the deep fascia halfway down the leg. The roof is pierced by the short saphenous vein.

1.57   BD

In the natal cleft, the sacral cornua are important surface markings for the sacral hiatus, through which a needle is passed for epidural anaesthesia. A direct inguinal hernia protrudes above and medial to the pubic tubercle. The external inguinal ring is palpable superolateral to the pubic tubercle. The femoral canal has the lacunar ligament as its medial wall. The ischial spine guides a needle to the pudendal canal for per vaginam pudendal nerve block. The transtubercular plane is an important landmark for lumbar puncture and transects the L5 vertebra (the supracristal plane, which passes through the L4 lumbar spine, can also be used).

1.58   ABCD

The scaphoid articulates with the radius, and since it transmits weight from the hand to the radial head it is commonly fractured during falls. When the fracture line severs the blood supply to the proximal fragment, avascular necrosis of the latter is a common complication. Tenderness in the anatomical snuffbox is initially the only clinical sign of the fracture before radiological evidence of osteonecrosis develops (2 weeks later). The flexor retinaculum takes its origin from the tubercle of the scaphoid and ridge on the trapezium. The adductor pollicis muscle has an origin from the capitate, not the scaphoid and so adduction of the thumb is unimpaired and pain-free after scaphoid fracture.

1.59   CDE

The dorsalis pedis artery lies between the extensor hallucis longus tendon medially, and the deep peroneal nerve lies laterally. The L5 dermatome lies over the medial half of the dorsum of the foot. The great saphenous vein is found anterior to the medial malleolus, and the lower limb of the extensor retinaculum passes under the medial longitudinal arch and blends with the plantar aponeurosis.

1.60   ABD

Sympathetic grey rami connect with all spinal nerve roots. The nervi erigentes originate from S2, S3 and often S4. The lumbosacral trunk (L4/5) passes anterior to the ala of the sacrum, under cover of the common iliac vessels, and joins the S1 ventral ramus above the piriformis muscle. The adductor muscles are supplied by the L2–L4 roots of the lumbar plexus. They develop by medial migration from the flexor (hamstring) compartment, and are therefore supplied by anterior divisions.

1.61   B

The thoracodorsal nerve is vulnerable in axillary surgery because of its unprotected prominence on the posterior wall. The whole of the serratus anterior muscle (eight costal digitations: one and two, into the superior angle; three and four, whole vertebral border; lower four, inferior angle) is used to protract the scapula, while the bulky insertion into the lower angle of the scapula aids the trapezius muscle in rotation. The long thoracic nerve (of Bell), which is protected underneath the fascia covering the serratus anterior muscle, innervates the muscle, originating from the C5–C7 roots.

1.62   All false

Flexion and extension take place between lumbar vertebrae, but the articular facets limit rotation. The left crus of the diaphragm is attached to the first two lumbar vertebrae. The iliolumbar ligament attaches to the lateral process of the L5 vertebra. At the level of the L3 vertebra the central canal contains the cauda equina. The iliolumbar branch of the posterior division of the internal iliac artery supplies the L5 vertebra. Only paired segmental lumbar branches of the abdominal aorta supply L1–L4 vertebrae.

1.63   BC

The antecubital fossa contains the posterior interosseous branch of the radial nerve (which leaves the fossa between the two heads of the supinator muscle) and the brachial artery (which lies lateral to the median nerve, against the tendon of the biceps muscle). The brachial artery bifurcates within the fossa into radial and ulnar arteries. Part of the roof is formed by the bicipital aponeurosis, which separates the superficial median cubital vein from the contents of the fossa. The brachioradialis and brachialis muscles and the medial edge of the supinator muscle form the floor.

1.64   AE

The carpal tunnel contains the median nerve, as well as the tendons of the flexor carpi radialis, flexor pollicis longus, and flexor digitorum alis superficialis and flexor digitorum profundus brevis tendons. The ulnar artery and nerve, and the flexor carpi ulnaris tendon, lie outside the tunnel. The flexor digitorum brevis muscle is found in the foot.

1.65   ADE

The superficial epigastric and superficial external pudendal arteries pass through the saphenous opening (the superficial circumflex and deep external pudendal arteries pierce the fascia lata). The femoral artery separates the femoral nerve (laterally) from the femoral vein (medially). The profunda femoris artery is a lateral branch of the femoral artery. The deep inguinal nodes lie medial to the femoral vein. The femoral sheath encloses the femoral vessels for up to 3 cm beyond the inguinal ligament, where the sheath terminates by fusing with the adventitia of both vessels.

1.66   AB

The patellar reflex is mediated by the femoral nerve formed from the posterior divisions of the L2–L4 anterior spinal rami, and is therefore lost after femoral nerve and L2–L4 dorsal root damage. T12 cord lesions result in an upper motor neurone lesion with exaggerated reflexes. Dorsal column lesions only affect central sensory processing since collaterals subserving spinal reflexes are preserved.

1.67   ACD

The musculocutaneous nerve (C5, C6) is a branch of the lateral cord of the brachial plexus and supplies the biceps. Each C5 and C6 spinal nerve is formed from dorsal (sensory) and ventral (motor) roots, mediating the afferent and efferent reflex arcs respectively. Each spinal nerve divides into a dorsal and ventral ramus. The C5 and C6 ventral rami form the upper trunk of the brachial plexus. The lateral cord is formed from anterior divisions of the upper (C5/C6) and middle (C7) trunks. So, neither the medial cord nor the middle trunk mediates the reflex.

1.68   All true

All muscles that insert into the extensor expansion extend the fingers at the interphalangeal joints. The lumbrical and interosseous muscles also flex the first metacarpophalangeal joints. The radial nerve is a branch of the posterior cord of the brachial plexus and innervates the long extensor muscles. The ulnar nerve supplies the two ulnar lumbrical muscles and all the interosseous muscles. The two radial lumbrical muscles are supplied by the palmar digital branches of the median nerve.

1.69   BE

The superficial palmar arch is incomplete over the thenar eminence. The radial artery passes over the dorsum of the wrist. The flexor digitorum superficialis tendons lie in the carpal tunnel medial to the median nerve and thenar eminence. All these structures therefore escape damage from a deep laceration into the thenar eminence. However, the recurrent branch of the median nerve and the adductor pollicis muscle would be involved, and so movements of the thumb would be restricted.

1.70   ABCD

Abduction of the arms is initiated by the supraspinatus muscle over the first 15°, and then continues to hold the head of the humerus against the glenoid cavity. The deltoid muscle then takes over and, at about 90°, the arm is laterally rotated, mainly by the infraspinatus muscle (both the supraspinatus and infraspinatus muscles stabilise the shoulder joint by tightening the rotator cuff). The scapula is then rotated by the combined actions of the trapezius and the inferior fibres of the serratus anterior muscles. The teres major muscle is a medial rotator and not part of the rotator cuff.

1.71   ACD

Nerve root involvement is suggested by pain radiating below the knee. It is worse when the nerve is stretched, as with the sciatic stretch test, or when intra-abdominal pressure is raised, as with straining at stool, coughing or sneezing. Urinary retention is a worrying sign but is not infrequently secondary to pain, analgesic medication and bedrest. Before this can be assumed, a full neurological examination must be performed; if there are concerns regarding a cauda equina syndrome, then further investigations must be carried out. An absent ankle jerk implies some nerve root damage, but on its own does not demand surgical intervention.

1.72   BDE

The piriformis muscle lies partly within the pelvis and emerges through the greater sciatic foramen to enter the gluteal region. The structures passing or emerging from the upper border of the piriformis muscle include the superior gluteal nerve and vessels. Below the lower border of the piriformis emerge the inferior gluteal nerve and muscles, pudendal nerve and vessels, the nerve to obturator internus and the sciatic nerve.

1.73   ACEF

The tibial nerve is the large terminal branch of the sciatic nerve. It runs through the popliteal fossa, at first lying on the lateral side, then crossing medial to the popliteal artery. It leaves the fossa by passing deep to gastrocnemius and soleus. The tibial nerve supplies the knee joint, popliteus, and the posterior compartment muscles of the leg and the foot.

1.74   ABEF

The IVC commences opposite the L5 vertebra, formed by the confluence of the right and left common iliac veins. It runs on the right of the aorta upwards towards the diaphragm and extends to the central tendinous diaphragm at the level of the body of the T8 vertebra. The IVC lies posterior to the bare area and caudate lobe of the liver. Due to its compound embryological origin, the tributaries are not identical to the branches of the abdominal aorta. On the right side, the testicular vein drains into the inferior vena cava; but on the left, the testicular vein drains into the left renal vein.

1.75   ADE

The middle meningeal artery divides from the maxillary branch of the external carotid, entering the cranium through the foramen spinosum. It is the largest artery that supplies the dura. While the maxillary artery does give off branches in the pterygopalatine fossa region, the middle meningeal artery comes off more proximally, deep to the ramus of the mandible.

1.76   AB

As soon as the aorta passes below the aortic hiatus, it gives off the coeliac plexus (T12). The plexus has three direct branches: left gastric, hepatic and splenic (mnemonic: left-hand side). The right gastric and gastroduodenal arteries are branches of the hepatic artery. The superior pancreatico-duodenal artery is a branch of the gastroduodenal artery.

1.77   EF

The right common carotid artery branches off the brachiocephalic artery. It bifurcates at the level of the upper border of the lamina of the thyroid cartilage. It lies posterior to the lobes of the thyroid gland and anterior to both the cervical sympathetic chain and the phrenic nerve on the scalenus anterior muscle; the latter is separated from the artery by prevertebral fascia.

1.78   ACDE

The basilic vein is a continuation of the ulnar stem of the dorsal venous arch in the hand. It lies medial to the biceps tendon in the cubital fossa and is medial to the medial cutaneous nerve of the forearm in the arm. The basilic vein ascends in the superficial fascia on the medial side of the biceps. It then pierces the deep fascia in the middle of the upper arm, is joined by the venae comitantes of the brachial artery, and becomes the axillary vein at the lower border of the teres major muscle.

1.79   ACDE

The popliteal artery divides into the anterior and posterior tibial arteries at the lower border of the popliteus muscle, anterior to the fibrous arch of the soleus muscle. The peroneal artery is the first branch of the posterior tibial artery. At the ankle joint, the posterior tibial artery passes deep to the flexor retinaculum.

1.80   ACF

The aorta enters the abdomen under the median arcuate ligament at T12 and divides into the common iliac arteries at L4 (intercristal plane). The cisterna chyli lies under cover of the right crus of the diaphragm, with the azygos vein on the right and the aorta to the left. In its course through the abdomen, the aorta gives off the three single ventral gut arteries (coeliac, superior and inferior mesenteric) and passes under the left renal vein. Unless the patient is obese, abdominal aortic pulsations are normally palpable.

1.81   ABCE

The surface marking of the femoral artery is the mid-inguinal point, which lies just medial to the position of the deep inguinal ring, which is at the midpoint of the inguinal ligament. The perforating branches of the profunda femoris artery supply the hamstrings. Branches of the circumflex femoral arteries contribute to the trochanteric anastomosis and feed the femoral head via their subretinacular branches. The femoral artery is subcutaneous in the femoral triangle, separated from skin by the fascia lata.

1.82   BCE

The portal vein is formed by the confluence of the superior mesenteric vein (lying to the right of the artery) and the splenic vein, behind the neck of the pancreas. It is about 5 cm long. The terminals of the portal vein and the hepatic artery form, with the hepatic ductules, the triads of the liver in the corners of the hexagonal lobules. The central veins drain into the hepatic veins.

1.83   AC

When the inferior thyroid arteries are ligated, the recurrent laryngeal nerves are vulnerable. When the superior thyroid arteries are ligated, the external laryngeal nerves running alongside could be damaged. The internal laryngeal nerves pass above and behind the root of the superior thyroid arteries and are therefore usually outside the operative field. The phrenic nerves are protected as they lie behind the prevertebral fascia. Both transverse cervical nerves run in the subcutaneous fascia. Horizontal skin-crease thyroidectomy incisions run parallel with their course, and therefore most branches of these cutaneous nerves are spared.

1.84   ABDE

The brachial artery begins at the lower border of the teres major muscle, terminating opposite the neck of the radius by branching into the radial and ulnar arteries. Its pulse can be palpated as it descends the arm overlapped by the medial border of the biceps muscle. The median nerve crosses over it (from lateral to medial), roughly before the artery's midpoint. In the upper arm the ulnar nerve travels alongside, lying posteriorly, but more distally it leaves the artery after piercing the medial intermuscular septum. The brachial artery is surrounded by venae comitantes, reinforced by the basilic vein. In the cubital fossa, the artery is overlain by the bicipital aponeurosis but it passes over the biceps tendon.

1.85   AC

The thoracic duct begins below the diaphragm as the cysterna chyli and then ascends through the aortic opening in the diaphragm, to the right of the descending aorta. It passes behind the oesophagus and then to the left of the oesophagus at the level of T5. It then runs upwards on the left side of the oesophagus into the neck. Here it crosses the subclavian artery to enter the left brachiocephalic vein. At the root of the neck, the thoracic duct receives the left jugular, subclavian and bronchomediastinal lymph trunks, although they may occasionally drain directly into the adjacent large vessels. The thoracic duct therefore conveys all the lymph from the lower limbs, pelvic cavity, abdominal cavity, left side of the thorax, head and neck and the left arm.

1.86   CEF

The function of lymphatic vessels is to return the plasma capillary filtrate to the circulation. This task is achieved by increased tissue pressure, facilitated by intermittent skeletal muscle activity, contractions of lymphatic vessels and an extensive system of one-way valves. Lymphoedema is an accumulation of tissue fluid resulting from a fault in the lymphatic system – very often, patients are diagnosed as having lymphoedema when the oedema is due to another cause. Lymphoedema can occur as a result of lymphatic obstruction secondary to infiltration of lymph nodes, frequently deep in the pelvis.

1.87   AB

The aorta enters the abdomen through the aortic hiatus of the diaphragm between the crura at the T12 level. The left lumbar veins pass behind it; anteriorly the aorta is related to the pancreas, which separates it from the stomach, the third part of the duodenum and mesentery of the small intestine. The aorta ends by dividing at the L4 level. Branches of the abdominal aorta are as follows:

- three unpaired anterior branches:
  - coeliac trunk
  - superior mesenteric artery (SMA)
  - inferior mesenteric artery (IMA)
- three lateral paired visceral branches:
  - adrenal
  - renal
  - gonadal
- five lateral paired parietal branches:
  - inferior phrenic
  - four pairs of lumbar arteries
- terminal branches:
  - common iliac arteries
  - median sacral artery.

The lumbar sympathetic trunk lies against the lumbar vertebral bodies. The left sympathetic trunk is overlapped by the abdominal aorta, and the right sympathetic trunk by the inferior vena cava.

1.88 ABCD

The vagus nerve travels in the carotid sheath in the neck. The sympathetic trunk lies alongside the cervical vertebrae, immediately behind the carotid artery, and has three cervical ganglia (superior, middle and inferior). During a left carotid endarterectomy (CEA), the thoracic duct may be seen. Pleural membranes are usually a little deeper and lateral to the site of CEA. The hypoglossal nerve passes forwards to supply the tongue and has to be protected, while the facial vein has to be ligated and divided to mobilise the internal jugular vein.

1.89 AB

The cephalic vein arises from the radial side of the dorsal venous arch of the hand and runs up the radial border of the forearm. It gives off a branch (the median cubital vein) in the cubital fossa and runs up the arm, lateral to the biceps. It lies anterior and lateral to the biceps tendon but never medial. The cephalic vein drains into the axillary vein. The axillary vein forms at the lower border of the teres minor where the basilic vein joins the venae comitantes of the brachial artery. It does contain valves.

1.90 ABC

The arch of the aorta commences from the manubriosternal joint and passes backwards over the left bronchus to reach the body of T4 vertebra just to the left of the midline. The arch is crossed on its left side by the phrenic and vagus nerves as they pass downwards in front of and behind the lung root, respectively. The left vertebral artery and the right internal mammary artery come off the left and right subclavian arteries, respectively.

1.91 ABC

As it leaves the cubital region, the radial artery passes medial to the biceps tendon, and superficial to the insertion of the pronator teres muscle. At the wrist, the artery passes across the floor of the anatomical snuffbox over the trapezium, and enters the hand between the two heads of the first dorsal interosseous and the oblique and transverse heads of the adductor pollicis muscles, continuing as the deep palmar arch. The arch is completed medially by a branch of the ulnar artery and allows for anastomosis between these two arteries.

1.92   ACDE
The submandibular gland is a lobulated gland made up of a superficial and a deep part, which are continuous with each other around the posterior border of the mylohyoid muscle. Part of the gland lies inferolaterally, enclosed in an investing layer of deep cervical fascia, platysma muscle and skin. Laterally it is crossed by the cervical branch of the facial nerve and vein. The facial artery is related to the posterior and superior aspects of the superficial part of the gland.

1.93   B
Three types of papillae are present on the upper surface of the anterior two-thirds of the tongue, namely: filiform, fungiform and (circum)vallate papillae. The mucous membrane covering the posterior one-third of the tongue is devoid of papillae but has a nodular irregular surface caused by the presence of underlying lymphatic tissue, the lingual tonsil.

1.94   BDE
The superior thyroid artery arises from the external carotid artery and enters the upper pole of the thyroid gland close to the external laryngeal nerve, which supplies the cricothyroid muscle, a tensor of the vocal cord. Damage to this nerve causes the loss of high-pitched phonation. The inferior thyroid artery, absent in 5%, arises from the thyrocervical trunk of the subclavian artery. The inferior thyroid artery should be ligated as far laterally as possible to avoid damaging the recurrent laryngeal nerve. Damage to one recurrent laryngeal nerve causes a weakened voice, damage to both causes semiadduction and respiratory difficulties. The isthmus is normally in front of the second and third tracheal rings, although variations are common.

1.95   ACE
The thyroid gland lies deep to the myofascial layer (strap muscles and investing layer of deep cervical fascia), closely applied to the thyroid and cricoid cartilages. The gland initially moves up on swallowing before returning to its normal position. The thyroid gland is highly vascular, normally accounting for 5% of cardiac output. While the superior thyroid artery is a branch of the external carotid artery, the inferior thyroid artery arises from the subclavian artery, via the thyrocervical trunk. There may also be a 'thyroidea ima' artery that may arise from the aortic arch, the brachiocephalic artery or even the internal mammary artery. The thyroid venous plexus usually drains via three pairs of veins: the superior and middle thyroid veins drain into the internal jugular; the inferior thyroid veins drain into the brachiocephalic vein.

1.96   BCEF

The sensory innervation to the tongue is from the VIIth, VIIIth and IXth cranial nerves. The tongue deviates to the side of a XIIth cranial nerve lesion on protrusion, is active during the first stage of swallowing and contains the lingual tonsil in the dorsum of its posterior third. The tongue is retracted up and back by the styloglossus muscle, protruded by genioglossus and depressed by the hyoglossus.

1.97   ABDF

The fibrous capsule of the parotid gland is an upward extension of the deep investing layer of cervical fascia that attaches to the zygomatic arch. The medial wall of the capsule is separated from the carotid sheath by the styloid process and associated muscles (stylopharyngeus, stylohyoid, styloglossus). The external carotid artery passes through the gland, supplying it as it does so. No facial vessels are related to the gland. The facial nerve enters the gland and divides within it into its five terminal branches.

1.98   CDE

The submandibular gland consists of a deep and a superficial part. The superficial part lies in the digastric triangle (above and between the two bellies of the digastric muscle). The hypoglossal nerve runs medial to the superficial part of the gland. The gland is superficial to the mylohyoid and hyoglossus muscles. A third of the submandibular gland lies below the lower border of the mandible and two-thirds above it.

1.99   DE

The true vocal folds have a stratified squamous epithelium, innervated by the recurrent laryngeal branch (CN X), and are formed by the vocal ligament (the free edge of the quadrangular membrane forms the false vocal cord). Above the vocal cords, the larynx is sensorily innervated by the internal laryngeal nerve (CN X). The cords are adducted by the lateral cricoarytenoid muscle, abducted by the posterior cricoarytenoid and tensed by tilting the thyroid cartilage downwards and forwards by contracting the cricothyroid muscle. All the laryngeal muscles are supplied by the recurrent laryngeal nerve except for cricothyroid, which is supplied by the external laryngeal nerve.

1.100   BC

The great auricular nerve turns upwards round the lateral border of the sternocleidomastoid muscle outside the triangle. The posterior belly of the omohyoid muscle and its intermediate tendon pass diagonally through the triangle (they are palpable, often confused with both the upper trunk of the brachial plexus and the suprascapular nerve), and the clavicular (intermediate) and acromial (lateral) branches of the supraclavicular nerves course through the roof. Lying medially, outside the triangle, are the roots of the brachial plexus, sandwiched between the scalenus posterior and medius muscles. The vertebral artery lies within the pyramidal space inferiorly, before ascending through the foramen transversarium of the C1–C6 vertebrae. Other components of the posterior triangle include the semispinalis capitis, splenius capitis, levator scapulae and scalenus medius muscles and the spinal accessory nerve.

1.101   AF

The axons conveying taste over the anterior two-thirds of the tongue and secretomotor fibres to the submandibular and sublingual salivary glands (the parotid is innervated by the IXth cranial nerve) are found in the chorda tympani nerve. The chorda tympani courses across the tympanic membrane beneath the mucous membrane of the middle ear after leaving the facial canal approximately 0.5 cm above the stylomastoid foramen. It exits the middle ear by passing through the petrotympanic fissure medially, and runs forwards on the medial side of the spine of the sphenoid bone. After entering the infratemporal fossa it merges with the lingual nerve. The chorda tympani, therefore, is not related to the parotid gland. It also escapes injury when the facial nerve is compressed within the most distal part of the facial canal. (The 'facial canal' is the passageway of the facial nerve after it emerges from the internal auditory meatus.)

1.102   ABCD

The pituitary fossa, or sella turcica, lies above the body of the sphenoid bone and its associated sinus. The pituitary fossa can be easily identified on a lateral skull X-ray. The optic chiasma lies above and towards the back of the sella turcica. A pituitary tumour would first impinge on the anterior part of the optic chiasma and so cause a temporal hemianopia.

1.103   C

The recurrent laryngeal nerves are sensory to the subglottic region and supply all the intrinsic muscles except the cricothyroid muscle.

1.104 B

The nasolacrimal duct drains into the inferior meatus; the sphenoidal air sinus drains into the sphenoethmoidal recess; and the posterior ethmoidal air sinus drains into the superior meatus. The middle meatus contains the bulla ethmoidalis of the middle ethmoidal air sinus, which drains through a hiatus in the bulla. Olfactory epithelium containing the primary olfactory neurones lines the superior nasal recess (roof of the nasal cavity) under cover of the cribriform plate of the ethmoid bone.

1.105 B

The posterior cerebral artery supplies the inferolateral surface of the temporal lobe, lateral and medial surfaces of the occipital lobe, the cerebral peduncle and the optic tract. Occlusion of this vessel results in a contralateral homonymous hemianopia.

1.106 CEG

The frontal nerve arises from the ophthalmic division of the trigeminal nerve in the lateral wall of the cavernous sinus. It enters the orbits through the superior orbital fissure. Just before it reaches the orbital margin it divides into the supratrochlear and supraorbital nerves. The supraorbital nerve passes through the supraorbital foramen, and supplies the skin of the forehead. The ophthalmic artery branches off the internal carotid artery at the cavernous sinus, and passes through the optic canal with the optic nerve. The optic nerve is surrounded by a sheath of pia, arachnoid and dura mater. The nasociliary nerve arises from the ophthalmic division of the trigeminal nerve in the lateral fourth of the cavernous sinus, and enters the orbit through the superior orbital fissure within the tendinous ring. The branches of the nasociliary nerve supply the ethmoidal sinuses, sphenoidal sinuses, skin of the upper eyelids and nose. The inferior ramus of the oculomotor nerve gives off branches to the inferior rectus, medial rectus and the inferior oblique muscles. The superior ramus of the oculomotor nerves supplies the levator palpebrae superioris, so may give rise to a ptosis if cut.

1.107 B

Earache from acute tonsillitis is due to referred pain along the glossopharyngeal nerve, which runs in the tonsillar bed and sends a tympanic branch to the tympanic plexus in the middle ear. The other nerves are not involved.

1.108 B
A right homonymous hemianopia would result from a left occipital lobe infarction and the macular would also be affected. Right eye blindness is seen when the right optic nerve is injured. The lateral rectus muscle is supplied by the VIth (abducent) cranial nerve, whose nucleus is in the caudal part of the pons.

1.109 ACE
The structures to be avoided at the time of submandibular gland excision include: the mandibular branch of the facial nerve; the hypoglossal and lingual nerves; and the facial artery and retromandibular vein. Lingual nerve damage results in ipsilateral anaesthesia and hemiplegia of the tongue. Hypoglossal nerve injury restricts the mobility of the tongue. Frey's syndrome (gustatory sweating) is a complication of parotid surgery.

1.110 DE
The anterior division of CN Vc has one sensory branch (the buccal nerve to the skin of the cheek and mucosa of the vestibule). All other branches are motor to the muscles of mastication (the masseter, temporalis and lateral pterygoid). The lower jaw teeth are supplied by the inferior alveolar branch of the posterior division of CN Vc. The buccinator muscle is supplied by the VIIth cranial nerve. Unopposed contraction of the contralateral lateral pterygoid muscle deviates the jaw to the side of the lesion during protrusion. None of the muscles of the pharynx are supplied by the anterior division of CN Vc, so dysphagia is not a feature of damage to this nerve.

1.111 CD
The head is turned using the contralateral sternocleidomastoid muscle, stimulated by impulses passing in the spinal accessory nerve. The movement takes place at the atlantoaxial joint about a vertical axis through the odontoid process of the axis, and is limited by the vertical alignment of the two attachments of the contralateral sternocleidomastoid muscle (contralateral mastoid process and sternoclavicular joint).

1.112 ABC

The optic nerve and retina are part of the central nervous system. The optic nerve is invested by all the meningeal layers. Since the central retinal artery travels in the optic nerve after branching off the ophthalmic artery, damage to the optic nerve commonly causes retinal infarction. Ptosis is a feature of both IIIrd nerve lesions and Horner's syndrome. The afferent arc of the corneal reflex is the nasociliary branch of CN Va. Blow-out fractures of the orbit either detach the suspensory ligament of the eye, or entrap the rectus muscles, usually the inferior rectus muscle; both conditions are associated with diplopia.

1.113 ACD

The transverse cervical nerve emerges as a single trunk behind the posterior border of the sternocleidomastoid and is superficial to the muscle. The transverse cervical artery is found in the posterior triangle of the neck just above the clavicle. The great auricular nerve (C2–C3) is a large trunk that passes vertically upwards over the sternocleidomastoid. The external jugular vein commences behind the angle of the mandible, formed by the union of the posterior auricular vein and the posterior division of the retromandibular vein. It descends obliquely across to the sternocleidomastoid and drains into the subclavian vein.

1.114 ABE

The inferior thyroid artery is a branch of the thyrocervical trunk, which arises from the subclavian artery. The inferior thyroid artery supplies the inferior pole of the thyroid gland and gives off oesophageal branches. In addition, it supplies both the superior and inferior parathyroid glands. The course of the inferior thyroid artery is closely related to the recurrent laryngeal nerve: in a thyroidectomy, therefore, it is preferable to ligate the artery lateral to the gland to avoid neural damage.

1.115 ABCE

The structures passing through the foramen magnum include: the medulla oblongata; meninges; spinal parts of the accessory nerves; meningeal branches of the upper cervical nerves; the vertebral arteries; and the anterior and posterior spinal arteries.

1.116   All true
The three compartments of the jugular foramen are: the anterior, containing the inferior petrosal sinus and the IXth cranial nerve; the middle, containing the Xth and XIth cranial nerves; and the posterior, containing the internal jugular vein as a continuation of the sigmoid sinus. The inferior petrosal sinus drains the cavernous sinus, leaving the skull via the jugular foramen and draining into the superior bulb of the internal jugular vein. The internal jugular descends the neck in the anterior of the carotid sheath, and drains into the brachiocephalic vein on each side behind the sternoclavicular joint. The ansa loops anteriorly around the carotid sheath under cover of the sternocleidomastoid muscle.

1.117   All false
The SVC drains all the structures above the diaphragm except the heart and lungs. It also receives the azygos vein, which drains the lumbar and subcostal regions. The SVC is formed behind the first costal cartilage by the union of the right and left brachiocephalic veins. It ends behind the third costal cartilage as it enters the right atrium. The SVC has no valves. The thoracic duct drains into the left brachiocephalic vein (or sometimes into the subclavian or internal jugular vein).

1.118   BCEF
The ophthalmic artery is a branch of the internal carotid and enters the orbit through the optic foramen. The ophthalmic artery then crosses the optic nerve to the medial side of the orbit accompanied by the nasociliary nerve. The supraorbital and nasal arteries are two branches of the ophthalmic artery that supply part of the skin of the forehead. The central retinal artery is the first and smallest branch of the ophthalmic artery. The cornea is avascular.

1.119   BD
The carotid artery divides into the external and internal carotid branches at the upper border of the thyroid cartilage. The external carotid artery is deep to the hypoglossal nerve, having been crossed by it at the level of the hyoid bone. The carotid sinus is normally found at the division of the common carotid artery or at the commencement of the internal carotid artery.

1.120   AB
The spinal canal is anterior to the ligamentum flavum but posterior to the vertebral disc. The spinal cord ends at L1.

1.121   AC

The thoracic duct leaves the cysterna chyli at the level of L1–L2, ascends into the thorax to the right of the descending thoracic aorta, crosses the midline gradually to reach the left border of the oesophagus (plane of Louis, T4), where it continues to run upwards, reaching the root of the neck. It then curves behind the carotid sheath and arches over the left subclavian artery to drain into the left brachiocephalic vein, although it can also drain into the other adjacent major veins. It carries lymph from the lower limbs, abdominal and pelvic regions, left thorax, left head and neck plus the left arm.

1.122   ADE

The eustachian tube in a child is shorter and more horizontal. The opening of the auditory tube lies above the soft palate adjacent to the tubal tonsil. The bony part of the eustachian tube perforates the petrous temporal bone.

1.123   ABD

A maldescended testis is one which has failed to reach the normal low position in the scrotum. Maldescent can be either arrested descent (cryptorchidism), where the testis is found at some point along the line of normal descent (intra-abdominal, inguinal canal, superficial inguinal pouch or high scrotum) or, less commonly, in a position not on the normal line of descent, that is ectopic (penile, superficial inguinal or femoral).

1.124   AD

The ischiorectal fossae, more accurately termed the 'ischioanal fossae', are wedge-shaped, fascia-lined spaces between the perianal skin and levator ani. The levator ani group is a thin muscular sheet with four groups of fibres: levator prostatae (men) or sphincter vaginae (women); puborectalis; pubococcygeus; and iliococcygeus. This group of muscles is supplied by S2–S4 roots. The levator ani also originates from the body of the pubis and the ischial spine. Whereas the aorta bifurcates at L4, the levator ani is found around the coccygeal level.

1.125 ABC

The superior mesenteric artery (SMA) supplies the entire small intestine except the proximal duodenum. The SMA also supplies the caecum, ascending colon and half the transverse colon. The origin of the SMA lies behind the neck of the pancreas (at L1 level). The SMA passes forwards and downwards in front of the uncinate process and the third part of the duodenum. Throughout, the superior mesenteric vein lies to its right. The splenic vein grooves the posterosuperior aspect of the pancreas and passes above the SMA.

1.126 ABCD

The epiploic foramen (of Winslow) is the communicating cavity between the greater and lesser sacs. It is an important surgical area, particularly for open cholecystectomy and gastrectomy. The lower boundary of the foramen is formed by the first part of the duodenum. The caudate lobe is the only part of the liver present in the lesser sac. It also forms the roof of the epiploic foramen. In the free edge of the lesser sac run the hepatic artery, portal vein and common bile duct.

1.127 AB

Hesselbach's triangle is the thin and weak part of the posterior wall of the inguinal canal, covered only by transversalis fascia and peritoneum, through which direct inguinal hernias arise. Its borders are the inferior epigastric artery, the inguinal ligament and the lateral border of the rectus abdominis muscle.

1.128 CE

The epiploic foramen (of Winslow) is the communicating cavity between the greater and lesser sacs. The caudate lobe of the liver forms the superior boundary. Anteriorly is the free border of the lesser omentum: its two layers containing the hepatic artery, common bile duct and portal vein. Posteriorly is the inferior vena cava, covered by peritoneum. Inferiorly is the first part of the duodenum (covered by peritoneum) and the hepatic artery. The gastroduodenal artery lies virtually anterior to the portal vein and is therefore anterior to the epiploic foramen. In Pringle's manoeuvre pressure is applied to the free edge of the lesser sac. This temporary manoeuvre is used to control major bleeding from a lacerated liver. The portal vein lies anterior to the common bile duct and the hepatic artery in this free edge.

1.129   AC
The psoas muscle has an origin from the transverse processes, bodies and intervertebral discs of T12–L5 and inserts along with the iliacus into the lesser trochanter. It is innervated by the lumbar plexus (L2–L4). The iliacus is supplied by the femoral nerve.

1.130   ABE
The body of the uterus is related anteriorly to the superior surface of the bladder or coils of small bowel. Posteriorly lies the pouch of Douglas. The body of the uterus is covered with peritoneum except where it is reflected off the bladder and at the broad ligaments. The uterine artery arises from the internal iliac artery and runs in the base of the broad ligament. The nerves of the uterus are derived from the inferior hypogastric plexus.

1.131   DE
The liver is mostly covered by peritoneum except for the bare area that lies to the right of the inferior vena cava between the coronary ligaments. The liver may be divided into eight anatomical segments. The right suprarenal gland (but not the left), kidney, right colic flexure, the duodenum and the gallbladder are in contact with the liver. The falciform ligament connects the liver to the anterior abdominal wall. The liver is largely separated from the diaphragm by the subphrenic recesses of the peritoneal cavity.

1.132   ABE
The territory of the mesenteric veins essentially follows that of their arteries. The inferior mesenteric vein drains the rectum via the superior rectal vein. The inferior mesenteric vein lies superficially, immediately below the peritoneum and to the left of the inferior mesenteric artery. After crossing over the left renal vein and under the body of the pancreas, it joins the splenic vein (the portal vein is formed downstream by the confluence of the splenic vein and superior mesenteric vein), though variations occur. Therefore, the superior mesenteric and splenic veins are considered tributaries of the portal vein, whereas the inferior mesenteric vein is not. The ileum is drained by the superior mesenteric vein as it is part of the mid-gut.

1.133 BDE
The portal vein is the confluence of the superior mesenteric vein after its union with the splenic vein. It lies in front of the inferior vena cava, and passes upwards behind the neck of the pancreas and first part of the duodenum. It runs in the free edge of the lesser omentum, forming the anterior boundary of the epiploic foramen. The portal vein receives tributaries from the left and right gastric, cystic and superior pancreatico-duodenal veins.

1.134 ABD
Both renal veins drain directly into the IVC. The left renal vein has further to travel and is therefore longer. The right suprarenal gland and right gonad have veins that drain directly into the IVC. The left suprarenal gland and left gonad drain into the left renal vein first. The IVC possesses a variable non-functioning valve at its orifice into the right atrium.

1.135 All true
Portal vein thrombosis may occur secondarily to thrombophilia or septic thrombophlebitis, possibly in severe appendicitis. It is one of the causes of small bowel infarction. It may result in portal hypertension, with small intestinal varices and splenomegaly.

1.136 BCDE
The sigmoid colon is supplied by the sigmoid branches of the inferior mesenteric artery. Sacral radicular branches are given off by the lateral sacral arteries and feed into the anterior and posterior spinal vessels of the sacral segments of the spinal cord. Both the trochanteric and cruciate anastomoses are fed by descending branches of the superior and inferior gluteal arteries, while the iliolumbar and superior gluteal arteries contribute to the anterior superior iliac spine anastomosis. The anterior division of the internal iliac artery supplies the bladder.

1.137 AD
Scrotal skin drains to the inguinal lymph nodes as does the distal end of the anal canal. The uterus drains mainly to the external iliac nodes but it is also possible for lymph to reach the inguinal nodes via the round ligament and inguinal canal. While lymph from the body of the uterus may reach the inguinal nodes, the cervix does not drain to the inguinal lymph nodes but to the external and internal iliac nodes that run in front of or behind the ureter. The cervix also drains to the sacral nodes via the uterosacral ligaments. The testes and fallopian tubes drain to the para-aortic nodes via lymphatics running back with the gonadal arteries.

1.138   ABCE

The superficial inguinal lymph nodes comprise a proximal group, below the inguinal ligament, and a distal group, lying alongside the termination of the great saphenous vein. The lateral nodes of the former group drain the buttock and back, and also the flank below the waist. The medial nodes drain the anterior abdominal wall below the umbilicus, including the external genitalia (excluding the testis), lower anal canal and perineum. The testes drain to the para-aortic nodes via lymphatics running back with the gonadal arteries. The fundus of the uterus drains via lymphatics accompanying the round ligament. The distal group of nodes drain superficial lymphatics from the lower limb.

1.139   CDE

Other relations include the left kidney and adrenal (not the right), the body and tail of the pancreas (not the head). The transverse mesocolon and the spleen are also relations.

1.140   ADE

Relations include the right and left bronchi, the trachea, the vagus nerve, pleura, the aortic arch and descending aorta and the thoracic duct.

1.141   CEF

Scarpa's fascia is divided in a Kocher's incision. T10 corresponds to the umbilical area. The rectus sheath is deficient posteriorly only below the arcuate line, but is present in two layers in the subcostal region.

1.142   ACE

The lienorenal ligament connects the hilum of the spleen to the left kidney. It contains both the splenic artery and vein as well as the tail of the pancreas. The left adrenal gland lies slightly above and behind the ligament.

1.143   C

On digital per-rectum examination, the structures that can be palpated in either sex are: the coccyx and lower sacrum behind; the ischial spines and ischiorectal fossae at the sides; and the anorectal ring at the anorectal junction. In men, the prostate can be felt (but normal seminal vesicles are not usually palpable). In women, the cervix can be felt through the vaginal wall, with the uterosacral ligaments laterally, and sometimes the ovaries.

1.144   AE

The epiploic foramen of Winslow lies behind the free edge of the lesser omentum. The posterior wall of the epiploic foramen is formed by the peritoneum of the posterior abdominal wall, which passes as a smooth layer from the hepatorenal pouch to the duodenum. Behind this peritoneum lies the inferior vena cava. The superior border of the epiploic foramen is formed by the inferior surface of the liver (caudate lobe). The first part of the duodenum forms part of the inferior border. The portal vein lies anteriorly in the free edge of the opening.

1.145   ACE

The first stem should not be confused with the suspensory ligaments of the breast, also known as the ligaments of Cooper. The duct of Santorini is the accessory pancreatic duct. The transversalis fascia and Scarpa's fascia are not related structures. Cloquet's node lies in the medial compartment of the femoral sheath where a small anatomical empty space exists and femoral hernias can occur. Alcock's canal is a fascial tunnel on the lateral wall of the ischiorectal fossa, which conveys the pudendal nerve and vessels.

1.146   ABC

The bare area of the liver is in direct contact with the right suprarenal gland and the diaphragm. The right suprarenal gland extends medially behind the IVC, separated from the 12th rib by the diaphragm. It typically has three arterial sources. It receives blood from the inferior phrenic artery, from a branch of the renal artery and from a branch directly from the aorta. The venous drainage is into the IVC by a very short vessel. The left suprarenal gland drains into its corresponding renal vein.

1.147   ACD

Scarpa's fascia is incised during the surgical approach to an inguinal hernia. The iliohypogastric nerve supplies the internal oblique and transversus, and may be divided during an appendicectomy, which may lead to a direct inguinal hernia. The iliohypogastric nerve is not encountered during normal inguinal hernia repair. However, the ilioinguinal nerve is usually seen. The nerve supplies cutaneous sensation to the skin at the base of the penis and part of the scrotum. Where it continues over the penis and scrotum, Scarpa's fascia assumes a different name: superficial perineal fascia of Colles. The superior epigastric vein drains the rectus muscle and enters the internal thoracic veins.

1.148 BE

The caudate lobe (segment I according to Couinaud's 1957 classification) lies posterior to the portal vein but anterior to the inferior vena cava. Three main hepatic veins divide the liver into four sectors, each of which receives a portal pedicle, with an alternation between hepatic veins and portal pedicles. According to this functional anatomy, the liver is divided into hemilivers (right and left) by the main portal scissura called Cantlie's line.

1.149 ACDE

The levator ani forms part of the deep external anal sphincter. The anal canal has no longitudinal muscular coat. Lymph from the lower anal canal drains via the superficial inguinal nodes. The entire anal sphincter is innervated by the inferior rectal branch of the pudendal nerve (S2–S4). The upper anal canal is thrown into vertical folds called anal columns. The anal valves are formed by horizontal semilunar folds of mucous membrane joining adjacent columns at their lower end. Anal valves are remnants of the proctodeal membrane. The anococcygeal body lies between the anal canal and the coccyx.

1.150 CD

The veins in the mesentery are all tributaries of the portal system. The root of the small bowel mesentery extends from a point to the left of the L2 vertebra, at the duodenojejunal junction, down to the right sacroiliac joint. The nerves are postganglionic sympathetic and preganglionic parasympathetic fibres (vagus nerve) from the superior mesenteric plexus. The superior mesenteric artery supplies the mid-gut, which includes the large bowel as far as the distal transverse colon. The transverse mesocolon lies anterior to the small bowel mesentery.

1.151 ABCE

The spleen lies on the diaphragm, separated from the ninth to 11th ribs by the costodiaphragmatic recess. The left extremity of the lesser sac extends into the hilum. The peritoneal fold known as the lienorenal ligament (which contains the splenic vessels and the tail of the pancreas touching the spleen) passes from the left kidney to the spleen. Another peritoneal fold, the gastrosplenic ligament, carries the short gastric and gastroepiploic vessels and joins the kidney to the stomach. The spleen is not palpable in the healthy individual, and must be enlarged by at least three times its normal size before it appears in the left hypochondrium.

1.152 ADF

In men, the deep perineal pouch contains the membranous urethra, sphincter urethra, bulbourethral glands, deep transverse perineal muscles, internal pudendal vessels and dorsal nerves of the penis. The bulb of the penis lies in the superficial perineal pouch.

1.153 E

The lower edge of the external oblique aponeurosis is folded back on itself between the anterior superior iliac spine (ASIS) and pubic tubercle, forming the inguinal ligament. The inguinal canal contains the ilioinguinal nerve (L1) and the genital branch of the genitofemoral nerve (L1–L2). The ilioinguinal nerve enters the inguinal canal via its anterior wall (not the deep ring) and runs outside the spermatic cord. The inferior epigastric artery marks the medial boundary of the deep inguinal ring. The deep inguinal ring is midway between the ASIS and pubic tubercle. Branches of the pudendal nerve (S2–S4) enter the perineum through the lesser sciatic foramen.

1.154 BCEG

The external (or superficial) inguinal ring is formed by a V-shaped defect in the external oblique aponeurosis above and medial to the pubic tubercle. It transmits the spermatic cord with all its contents, plus the ilioinguinal nerve. The following are the contents of the spermatic cord: three fascial layers (external spermatic, cremasteric, internal spermatic); three arteries (testicular, cremasteric, artery to the vas deferens); the pampiniform plexus, veins from the cremaster and vas deferens; and the genital branch of the genitofemoral nerve, sympathetic fibres, vas deferens and lymphatics.

1.155 AB

Rupture of the spongy (penile) part of the urethra leaks urine into the superficial perineal fascia (of Colles), which is continuous with the membranous fascia (of Scarpa) in the anterior abdominal wall. The penile urethra takes a 90° angle through the bulbar part. The corpus spongiosum invests the penile urethra.

1.156 DEF

Ejaculatory ducts enter the upper posterior part of the prostate gland to open into the urethra. Laterally lies the levator ani. The arterial supply to the prostate is derived from the inferior vesical artery, a branch entering the prostate at each side. The prostate is surrounded by a venous plexus, which drains into the internal iliac vein and subsequently into the internal vertebral venous plexus.

1.157   CD
The posterior third of the tongue has no papillae but does contain the lingual (lymphoid) tonsil. The mucous membrane of the posterior third of the tongue is innervated by the IXth cranial nerve for both general and taste sensations. The very posterior of the dorsum of the tongue is innervated by the internal laryngeal nerve, a branch of the superior laryngeal nerve (CN X). The chorda tympani (CN VII) is the nerve for taste to the anterior two-thirds of the tongue.

1.158   ADEF
The ilioinguinal nerve (L1) emerges laterally to the psoas, descends posterior to the kidney and enters the inguinal canal by piercing the transversus abdominis and internal oblique muscles (not by passing through the deep ring). It then leaves the inguinal canal via the superficial inguinal ring. It is sensory to the skin of the lower abdomen and some of the genital area. The ilioinguinal (and iliohypogastric) nerves carry motor fibres to the external and internal obliques and the transversus abdominis. They travel in the anterior abdominal wall between the transversus and internal oblique muscles close to McBurney's point – so if they are damaged after a grid-iron incision, the muscle fibres in the conjoint tendon will be paralysed and this may give rise to an indirect inguinal hernia.

1.159   DE
The rectum contains no mesentery by definition, although parts are covered by peritoneum. The pararectal lymph nodes drain into the inferior mesenteric and internal iliac nodes. The superior rectal vein drains into the inferior mesenteric vein (portal circulation). The middle rectal vein drains into the internal iliac vein and the inferior rectal vein drains into the internal pudendal vein (both systemic circulation). The arterial supply is principally from the superior rectal artery with contributions from the middle and inferior rectal and median sacral vessels.

1.160   ABCD
The kidneys lie retroperitoneally in the upper posterior abdominal wall. They are mostly covered by the costal margin. Both kidneys are in contact posteriorly with the costodiaphragmatic recess, psoas muscle, subcostal and ilioinguinal nerves. The cisterna chyli is found on the right of the aorta in front of L1 and L2. It is at a similar level to the kidneys and lies between them without direct contact.

1.161   A

The femoral artery enters the thigh halfway between the anterior superior iliac spine and the pubic symphysis. Here the femoral artery lies on the psoas major tendon, which separates it from the capsule of the hip joint. The femoral artery emerges from the femoral canal and then courses downwards to disappear beneath the sartorius, entering the adductor canal. Only the profunda femoris spirals deep to the adductor longus. At the adductor hiatus, the femoral vein is lateral but ascends posteriorly in the canal until it reaches the femoral triangle, where it lies medial to the femoral artery. The femoral artery gives off a descending genicular artery while in the adductor canal.

1.162   ABE

The sural nerve branches off the tibial nerve in the popliteal fossa. It is usually joined by the sural communicating branch of the common peroneal nerve and supplies the back of the leg and the lateral foot. The tibial nerve enters the popliteal fossa lateral to the popliteal artery and then passes posterior then medial to the artery. Damage to the tibial nerve results in loss of plantar flexion of the feet. The tibial nerve is superficial to both popliteal vein and artery in the popiteal fossa.

1.163   ABEFG

The linea semilunaris marks the lateral margin of the rectus muscle and sheath, passing from the pubic tubercle to the costal cartilage at the tip of the ninth rib, which overlies the fundus of the gallbladder on the right. The inferior epigastric vessels and medial umbilical ligament cross the linea posteriorly below the arcuate line, before ascending in the posterior compartment of the rectus sheath. The anterior abdominal wall would be greatly weakened both physically and functionally by cutting along the semilunar line as the nerve supply to the rectus abdominis muscle and overlying skin would be interrupted. Furthermore, Langer's lines on the abdomen are horizontal. Spigelian hernias occur at the edge of the linea semilunaris, typically at the level of the arcuate line. The three borders of Hesselbach's triangle are the inferior epigastric artery, the inguinal ligament and the lateral border of the rectus abdominis muscle (linea semilunaris).

1.164   E
From superficial to deep, the scalp has five basic layers, denoted by the mnemonic 'SCALP': skin; connective tissue; aponeurosis; loose areolar tissue; and periosteum. The blood supply to the scalp is from branches of both the internal and external carotid arteries. Two such tributaries from the internal carotid are the supraorbital and supratrochlear arteries. There is no C1 dermatome. The aponeurosis of the scalp is separated from the epicranium by loose connective tissue (the plane of cleavage in scalping), facilitating gliding movements. It contains no lymph nodes. Lymphatic drainage is mainly to the submandibular, preauricular, mastoid and occipital nodes. The occipitofrontalis muscle is supplied by the VIIth cranial nerve.

1.165   ACE
The third part of the duodenum lies in the subcostal plane (L3) and follows the inferior margin of the pancreatic head. The third part of the duodenum lies posterior to the superior mesenteric vessels. It overlies the aorta and the beginning of the inferior mesenteric artery. The root of the small bowel mesentery is attached near its termination on the left. The second part of the duodenum overlies the right ureter and renal vessels in the hilum of the right kidney, separated from the renal artery by the vein.

1.166   BD
The head of the pancreas is related to the hilum but does not overlie the right kidney. It is, however, anterior to the left kidney. The transpyloric plane (L1) transects the pancreas obliquely, passing through the midpoint of the neck, with most of the head below the plane, and most of the body and tail above. The transverse mesocolon is attached to the head, neck and body of the pancreas. The uncinate process lies posterior to the superior mesenteric vessels, and the inferior mesenteric vein passes behind the body of the pancreas, where it joins the splenic vein.

1.167   AC
The medial plantar nerve is a branch of the tibial nerve and supplies the medial three and a half toes on the plantar surfaces and the dorsal surfaces proximal to the nailbeds. The medial branch of the superficial peroneal nerve partly supplies the skin of the medial big toe and adjacent parts of the second and third toes.

1.168   ABD
The jejunum has a thicker wall, less mesenteric fat, more plicae circulares, a wider lumen, fewer Peyer's patches and fewer arterial arcades than the ileum.

1.169   ABC
The spermatic cord contains three fascial layers (external spermatic, cremasteric, internal spermatic) and three arteries (testicular, cremasteric, artery to the vas deferens). Other structures include: pampiniform plexus, vas deferens, the genital branch of the genitofemoral nerve, sympathetic fibres and lymphatics. The ilioinguinal nerve enters the inguinal canal but not the spermatic cord.

1.170   CDE
The medial ligament of the ankle, otherwise known as the 'deltoid ligament', has two layers. The deep part is narrow and much shorter than the superficial part, which is triangular in shape. The superficial part of the medial ligament is attached to the borders of the tibial malleolus, and has a continuous attachment from the medial tubercule of the talus along the edge of the sustentaculum tali and spring ligament to the tuberosity of the navicular bone. The lateral ligament consists of three separate bands, and it is this ligament which is usually damaged in inversion injuries (a sprain) of the ankle. The ligaments themselves cannot be seen on X-ray, although avulsion fractures may be detectable on X-ray.

1.171   BCD
The IVC commences opposite the L5 vertebra. It runs on the right side of the aorta, upwards beyond the aortic opening of the diaphragm and extends to the central tendon of the diaphragm, which it pierces at the level of T8. The IVC lies behind the portal vein near the pancreas and bile duct, and forms the posterior wall of the epiploic foramen of Winslow. The right vein of the suprarenal gland is usually only a few millimetres long and enters the IVC directly. The left suprarenal vein is longer and enters the left renal vein.

1.172   D

The processus vaginalis is a parietal peritoneal sac which passes through the internal ring of the inguinal canal in the fetus, but which is normally obliterated after birth except for a small part that becomes the tunica vaginalis of the testis. The testis descends through the canal as a retroperitoneal structure and is therefore outside and behind the processus vaginalis. In cases of a persistent processus vaginalis, indirect inguinal hernias can ensue.

1.173   BDE

The adductor canal (also known as the subsartorial or Hunter's canal) is a 15-cm long tunnel bounded by vastus medialis laterally, and adductor longus and magnus posteriorly. The canal serves as a passage for the superficial femoral artery, femoral vein, saphenous nerve and the nerve to vastus medialis to pass into the popliteal fossa. The adductor canal begins where the sartorius crosses over the adductor longus and ends at the adductor hiatus. The femoral artery gives off a descending genicular artery while in the adductor canal. The nerve to the tensor fascia lata is the superior gluteal nerve (L4–S1), which passes through the greater sciatic foramen.

1.174   D

Ribs are narrow, flat, curved bones that form the thoracic cage. The rib has an angle at its posterior end. The costal groove is found on the inferior border of the ribs. The intercostal vessels and nerve run in this groove. Ribs typically articulate with their corresponding vertebra plus the one above it. The area just anterior to the angle is the weakest, and therefore the most likely to fracture in trauma.

1.175   AC

The axillary artery commences at the lateral border of the first rib and is a continuation of the subclavian artery. The axillary artery becomes the brachial artery at the inferior border of teres major. The axillary artery can be divided into three parts by the pectoralis minor. In its first part, it gives off the superior thoracic artery; in the second part, the thoraco-acromial and lateral thoracic arteries; and in the third part, the subscapular, anterior and posterior circumflex arteries.

1.176   BCDE

The right and left gastric arteries supply the lesser omentum as they lie between its two peritoneal layers. The free edge of the lesser omentum is attached to the first 2 cm of the first part of the duodenum below and the fissure of the ligamentum venosum above. The common hepatic duct is joined by the cystic duct to form the common bile duct in the free edge of the lesser omentum. The greater omentum is quite mobile.

1.177   BCD

The subclavian artery is closely related to the brachial plexus, the phrenic and vagus nerves (and recurrent laryngeal nerve on the right side only). The stellate ganglion is deeper within the neck and the thoracic duct lies on the left side. The approach to the subclavian artery may be supraclavicular and involve removal or division of the clavicle, dissection of the scalenus anterior, pectoralis major and pectoralis minor muscles.

1.178   ACDEF

Most of the anterior surface of the uterus is applied to the posterior surface of the bladder. Ureteric calculi are palpable through the posterior fornix, lateral to the cervix, where the ureter passes under the uterine artery ('water under the bridge'). Lymphatic drainage of the medial part of the fallopian tubes and uterine fundus is via the lymphatics in the broad ligament to the superficial inguinal nodes. The main arterial supply of the uterus is from the uterine artery, a branch of the internal iliac. The round ligament is a gubernacular remnant.

1.179   ACDE

Parasympathetic fibres supply the main motor innervation of the bladder via the pelvic splanchnic nerves (S2–S4). Sympathetic fibres come from L1–L2 via the superior hypogastric and pelvic plexuses. The external sphincter contains skeletal muscle and is supplied by the perineal branch of the pudendal nerve (S2–S4). The obturator nerve, which is a branch of the lumbar plexus, is formed within the substance of psoas major from the anterior divisions of L2–L4 and supplies some parietal peritoneum and skin on the medial side of the thigh.

1.180   ADE

The 'important' cortical areas of the temporal lobe area are the auditory cortex and temporal association area (responsible for the recognition of auditory stimuli and integration with other modalities). Cerebral abscesses act as space-occupying lesions and produce focal neurological deficits. They may also cause meningitis, epilepsy and intracranial herniation.

1.181   A

The superficial venous network (dorsal venous arch) on the dorsum of the hand drains partly into the cephalic vein just distal to the anatomical snuffbox. The cephalic vein then winds around onto the anterolateral aspect of the forearm. It runs in the upper arm lateral to the biceps in the deltopectoral groove and perforates the clavipectoral fascia to drain into the axillary vein. The axillary vein is formed by the union of the vena comitantes of the brachial artery and the basilic vein at the lower border of the teres major muscle.

1.182   BCD

The medial wall, which separates the middle from the internal ear, contains the oval window and promontory. The promontory is the rounded projection of the first turn of the cochlea. Also medially, the internal auditory meatus carries the facial nerve. The floor is a thin bone separating the middle ear from the bulb of the jugular vein. Anteriorly, a thin bony wall separates the cavity from the internal carotid artery.

1.183   DE

The palatine tonsil lies in the oropharynx, in a pit floored by the superior constrictor muscle, through which the IXth cranial nerve passes. The tonsil is supplied by the tonsillar branch of the facial artery. Venous blood first drains into the tonsillar venous plexus, then into the pharyngeal venous plexus and thence into the external palatine vein (a bleeding point after tonsillectomy), or the facial and pharyngeal veins.

1.184   All true

The ischiorectal fossae, more accurately termed 'ischioanal fossae', are wedge-shaped, fascia-lined spaces between the perianal skin and levator ani. Infection from one fossa may spread across the midline through the retrosphincteric space of the anococcygeal raphe posteriorly, but the anterior recesses, which extend above the perineal membrane, remain separate. The base of each fossa is formed by skin and superficial fascia and may be easily incised to drain ischiorectal abscesses. The inferior rectal nerves and internal pudendal vessels are not usually damaged since they arch high in the roof.

1.185   All false
The sciatic nerve appears in the gluteal region below the lower border of the piriformis muscle in the vast majority of cases, deep to the lower medial quadrant, and lateral to the inferior gluteal vessels. In its descent, it is separated from the capsule of the hip joint anteriorly by the obturator internus tendon, and by the gemelli muscles.

1.186   ABDE
The recurrent laryngeal nerves arise from the vagus. On the right, the recurrent laryngeal nerve winds around the subclavian artery; on the left, it winds around the aortic arch, passing behind the ligamentum arteriosum. Both nerves run in a groove between the trachea and oesophagus and are closely related to the inferior thyroid artery.

1.187   ABD
Each renal artery usually divides into five segmental branches before entering the renal pelvis. It supplies the ureter and lies posterior to the renal vein, but anterior to the renal pelvis. After branching off the aorta, the renal artery passes in front of the inferior vena cava.

1.188   ACE
The major arterial supply to the ureter is (from superior to inferior): the renal artery, the gonadal artery and the superior vesical artery. The blood supply to the ureter is reinforced at intervals by small branches of the lumbar arteries. The ureter lies posterior to the gonadal vessels and vas, but descends anterior to the psoas muscle and the bifurcation of the common iliac artery.

1.189   ABDE
The popliteus tendon penetrates the capsule and is covered by synovial membrane. The suprapatellar bursa, although developing as an isolated cavity, later fuses with the joint space. The iliotibial tract is attached to a smooth round facet on the anterolateral aspect of the lateral condyle of the tibia. The middle geniculate artery pierces the joint capsule to supply it and the cruciate ligaments. Flexion occurs in the upper compartment and rotation in the lower compartment of the knee.

1.190   BCD

The trigeminal (V) nerve has sensory fibres to the greater part of the skin of the face, mucous membranes of the mouth, nose and paranasal air sinuses. It provides motor innervation to the muscles of mastication (temporalis, masseter, pterygoid). The buccinator muscle is supplied by the facial nerve. The angle of the mandible is supplied by the great auricular nerve (C2–C3).

1.191   BD

Cervical rib is present in about 0.5% of the population, of which 60% are symptomatic. Symptoms due to the presence of a cervical rib depend on the structure it is compressing. Neurological symptoms are the most common presentation, usually compression of the C8 and T1 nerve roots, which causes pain and paraesthesiae on the ulnar aspect of the arm and forearm and wasting of the small muscles of the hand. Vascular changes are seen less often. The arm can become swollen as a result of venous compression. Compression of the subclavian artery can lead to thrombus formation, emboli, ischaemic changes, and even gangrene.

1.192   All true

The base of the bladder is its posterior surface and is triangular. On the base of the bladder in men, the vas deferens lies uppermost and loops medially over the ureters ('water under the bridge'), which separate the seminal vesicle from the vas. In women, the cervix and anterior vaginal wall are attached to the base of the bladder.

1.193   ABD

The posterior relations of the right kidney are the diaphragm, quadratus lumborum, psoas, transversus abdominis, the 12th rib on the right, and the 11th and 12th ribs on the left. Furthermore, the posterior recess of the pleura lies posteriorly as does the subcostal vein, artery and nerve (T12), and the ilioinguinal (L1) and iliohypogastric (L1) nerves. The suprarenal gland lies superomedial to the kidney.

1.194 AB

The thyroid gland has a definite, fine capsule, which allows a capsular dissection to preserve the recurrent laryngeal nerves. The superior parathyroid glands are more constant in position than the inferior. Because of their embryological migration, the inferior glands may be situated among the pretracheal lymph nodes or in the thymus as far as 10 cm from the thyroid. The middle thyroid veins are the least constant of the thyroid veins. The superior veins drain into the internal jugular vein; the inferior veins are very constant and drain into the brachiocephalic veins; and the middle veins are very variable and often multiple. Unilateral recurrent laryngeal nerve section results in the ipsilateral vocal cord lying motionless in the mid- or cadaveric position. The voice is hoarse and weak. If both recurrent laryngeal nerves are divided, then the glottic space is narrowed and stridor develops.

1.195 ABE

In Horner's syndrome there is: ptosis, pupillary constriction and occasional enophthalmos, and dryness and flushing of the skin of the head and neck. The sympathetic supply to the lungs is preserved as this originates below the lesion directly from the T1–T4 ganglia of the sympathetic chain. Sympathetic fibres pass to the arm via grey rami from the middle and inferior cervical sympathetic ganglia through all the roots of the brachial plexus.

1.196 BCDE

The trachea commences just below the cricoid cartilage (at the level of C6). Within the thorax and on the right, the trachea is in contact with the pleura, vagus and subclavian artery. On its left, the trachea is in contact with the left recurrent laryngeal nerve, aortic arch and the left common carotid and subclavian arteries. The trachea ends at the upper border of T5, where it bifurcates.

1.197 All false

The prostate is an inverted cone, so it has a base in contact with the bladder neck above it and an apex lying against the urogenital diaphragm below it. The seminal vesicles drain into the vas deferens posterior to the bladder to form the common ejaculatory ducts, which pierce the prostate and empty into the prostatic urethra. The prostatic venous plexus lies outside the capsule and therefore 'shelling' of the prostate from inside the capsule is a relatively avascular procedure. The prostate is separated from the rectum by the rectovesical fascia (of Denonvilliers).

1.198   ABCE
The pituitary sits in the sella turcica of the sphenoid. It is covered by the diaphragma sellae (fold of dura) which separates it from the optic chiasma above. There is an opening in the diaphragma for the pituitary stalk. The cavernous sinuses are found laterally and the sphenoid sinuses inferiorly.

1.199   C
The lateral malleolus is grooved by the peroneus brevis tendon; the medial malleolus by the tibialis posterior tendon. The superficial part of the deltoid ligament is attached to the sustentaculum tali of the calcaneus. Posterior to the medial malleolus, the tibial nerve lies posterior to the posterior tibial artery, and these lie between the flexor hallucis longus tendons posteriorly, and the flexor digitorum longus tendons anteriorly.

1.200   DE
When a right hemicolectomy is performed, the gonadal vessels are encountered first and then the second part of the duodenum and right ureter. It is wise to clearly identify the ureter, although formal dissection and display is not always needed.

1.201   BC
The pharyngotympanic tube drains the middle ear into the nasopharynx by piercing the pharyngobasilar fascia. The cartilaginous part gives attachment to the tensor veli palatini muscle. It opens on swallowing under the action of the salpingopharyngeus and tensor palati muscles, and is obstructed by an enlarging pharyngeal tonsil (adenoids).

1.202   ABD
The facial nerve gives off a branch to the stapedius before it enters the stylomastoid foramen. The buccinator is supplied by the buccal branches of the facial nerve. The medial (and lateral) pterygoid is supplied by the mandibular division of the trigeminal nerve. The parasympathetic supply to the lacrimal gland is from the secretomotor fibres from the superior salivatory nucleus travelling in the intermediate and greater petrosal nerves and relaying in the pterygopalatine ganglion. The parasympathetic supply to the parotid gland is from the inferior salivatory nucleus via the tympanic and lesser petrosal branches of the glossopharyngeal nerve that project to the otic ganglion (preganglionic). Postganglionic fibres pass from the otic ganglion to the parotid via the auriculotemporal nerve.

1.203   CD

All joints in the body can be broadly divided into three types: fibrous, cartilaginous (primary and secondary) and synovial (typical and atypical). Primary cartilaginous joints are formed when the bone meets (joins) a cartilage. They are quite immobile and very strong. The adjacent bone may fracture but the bone–cartilage interface seldom separates. All epiphyses and the ribs attaching to their costal cartilages are examples of primary cartilaginous joints. Fibrous joints unite the bones of the vault of the skull at the sutures. The bone ends are simply joined by fibrous tissue and the movement is negligible. A secondary cartilaginous joint is a union between bones whose articular surfaces are covered with a thin lamina of hyaline cartilage, which in turn is frequently united by fibrocartilage. All midline joints – symphysis pubis, sternal angle, xiphisternum and intervertebral discs – are examples of secondary cartilaginous joints.

In a synovial joint, the bone ends are covered by hyaline cartilage and surrounded by a capsule, enclosing a joint cavity. The capsule is lined internally by synovial membrane (containing synovial fluid) and the capsule is reinforced internally or externally, or both, by ligaments. The joint is capable of varying degrees of movement. All limb joints fall into this category. In atypical synovial joints, such as the sternoclavicular joint and the acromioclavicular joint, there is no hyaline cartilage in the joint. The cartilaginous epiphysis, like all hyaline cartilage, has no blood supply. The synovial membrane, joint mesenchyme and its derivatives are supplied from a vascular plexus that surrounds the epiphysis and sends branches to the joint structures. As ossification of the cartilaginous epiphysis begins, branches from this vascular circle penetrate the ossification centre.

1.204   BCE

The knee joint is a synovial and a hinge joint. The capsule of the knee joint is thin anteriorly and posteriorly but reinforced on either side by strong collateral ligaments. Both the anterior and posterior cruciate ligaments are intracapsular, but extrasynovial. The medial and lateral menisci are C-shaped, with their anterior and posterior horns attached to the intercondylar eminence of the tibia and their outer borders to the joint capsule. The meniscofemoral ligament is adjacent to the posterior cruciate ligament and attaches the posterior border of the lateral meniscus close to the femoral attachment of the posterior cruciate ligament. It stabilises the meniscus during rotation of the femur on the tibia. The oblique popliteal ligament is a lateral expansion from the insertion of semimembranosus which slopes up to the popliteal surface of the femur. The obliquity of this ligament limits rotation-extension in the 'screw-home' or locked position.

The anterior cruciate ligament, running upwards and backwards from the anterior part of the tibial plateau towards the lateral condyle of the femur, prevents backward displacement of the femur on the tibial plateau. It also limits extension of the lateral condyle of the femur which then causes medial rotation of the femur in the 'screw-home' position of full extension. The posterior cruciate ligament, running obliquely from the posterior part of the tibia towards the medial condyle of the femur, prevents the femur from sliding forwards off the tibial plateau. In the weight-bearing, flexed knee it is the only stabilising factor for the femur and its attached quadriceps. The suprapatellar bursa is continuous with the synovial cavity of the joint, and therefore it provides a route for injecting or withdrawing fluid into or from the joint. After injuries to the joint, fluid accumulates (effusion) in the suprapatellar bursa, causing typical fullness around the knee. The pre- and infrapatellar bursae, however, do not communicate with the joint.

1.205   BE
L5 cord lesions cause an ipsilateral loss of fine touch and a contralateral loss of pain and temperature sensation below the lesion. There is an ipsilateral upper neurone lesion, with brisk reflexes, a Babinski sign, but no muscle wasting.

1.206   AD
Lateral swellings of the neck include lymph nodes, salivary glands, branchial cysts, cervical ribs, carotid body tumours (chemodectomas), cystic hygromas, sternocleidomastoid tumours, arteriovenous fistulae and lateral thyroid lobe lesions.

1.207   BC
Swellings of the neck considered to be midline include thyroglossal cysts, pharyngeal pouches, plunging ranulae, subhyoid bursae, laryngoceles and lesions in the thyroid isthmus.

SECTION 2: PHYSIOLOGY – ANSWERS

2.1   AC
During exercise cardiac output increases sixfold (stroke volume × 2 and heart rate × 3). There is usually no change in PaO_2 and $PaCO_2$. An increase in systolic and a decrease in diastolic pressure is seen. Renal blood flow is reduced and there is an increase in negative intrathoracic pressure.

2.2   ACD
$PaCO_2$ is often lowered in severe exercise. The increase in ventilation is probably due to a neural drive to the respiratory centre, together with a voluntary drive to contracting muscles. The stroke volume increases twofold, the ventilatory rate 15-fold and the heart rate threefold; the blood pressure also rises. The relationship between heart rate and O_2 consumption is linear. There is approximately a twofold increase in oxygen consumption, therefore the mixed venous blood O_2 saturation falls to 50%.

2.3   ACE
During the acute phase of injury, the body enters a catabolic phase in which increased levels of catecholamines cause glycogen to be broken down in the liver and muscle to provide glucose. Insulin levels fall and the glucose levels rise. Increased sympathetic activity also causes mobilisation of fat from adipose tissue.

2.4   BCD
Cardiac muscle is unable to regenerate, and therefore scar tissue is formed following myocardial infarction. Peripheral nerves regenerate following injury, and growth is said to occur at a rate of 1 mm/day. Schwann cells are responsible for the myelination of peripheral nerves: these cells are involved in peripheral nerve regeneration through the production of growth factors as well as in forming growth channels for new nerve axons. Renal tubules (cortical) do not regenerate following injury.

2.5   D
Body water content is 60% in the adult male and this equates to about 45 litres. Neonates comprise 75% water. The plasma volume measures about 3.5 litres and the total blood volume is around 5 litres. Approximately 400 ml of water is lost daily from the lungs. The intracellular fluid is about two-thirds of total body water, that is 30 litres out of a total body water content of 45 litres. Daily potassium requirements are approximately 1 mmol/kg. The normal serum potassium concentration is around 3.5–5.0 mmol/l.

2.6   BC

Collagen provides the tensile strength, whereas elastin provides elasticity. Together they make the skin tough, flexible and deformable, but with the property of returning to its original shape once the deforming stresses are released. Type I collagen predominates during the maturation stage of wound healing. Initially, type III predominates. Collagen remodelling occurs at around 14 days. Various factors can impair healing and repair: age, disorders of nutrition (zinc, vitamin C deficiency), neoplastic disorders, Cushing's syndrome and steroid therapy, diabetes mellitus and immunosuppression, vascular disturbance and denervation.

2.7   BE

A sutured, clean surgical wound heals by primary intention. Open wounds heal by secondary intention. Fibroblasts produce collagen and extracellular matrix. Myofibroblasts are the cells responsible for wound contracture. Steroids, azathioprine, diabetes mellitus, vitamin C and zinc deficiencies all delay wound healing. Hyperbaric oxygen is being used in some centres for cases of gas gangrene (as oxygen is toxic to anaerobes) but has not been proved to significantly accelerate wound healing, although it may help if there is an ischaemic element.

2.8   AB

Hypertrophy is the increase in size of a tissue due to the increase in size of the cells present. It is reversible if the stimulus is removed. An increase in cell number is called hyperplasia. Mitosis is the means by which cells divide and increase in number (cell division).

2.9   ABCD

The GFR varies during life. Adult levels are reached at 2 years of age and decline linearly from 40 years due to glomerular sclerosis. In research laboratories, GFR can be measured by inulin clearance. Inulin is a polymer of fructose that is not secreted, metabolised or reabsorbed by the kidney. This means that the amount of inulin excreted in urine (per minute) equals the amount of inulin filtered at the glomerulus (per minute). In clinical practice, GFR is estimated by measuring the creatinine clearance. A 50% increase in GFR occurs during pregnancy. GFR increases after a protein-rich meal.

2.10   BC

Wounds of the skin, subcutaneous tissues, muscle, fascia and tendon only ever regain 80–90% of their pre-injury strength. The development of wound strength depends on the type of collagen produced. Type III collagen is produced during the early phase of wound healing, and is weaker than the later-appearing type I collagen (maturation stage). The process of skin healing includes a lag phase lasting 1–2 weeks after the injury, followed by a proliferative phase lasting 2–12 weeks, and finally a scar maturation phase lasting from months to years.

2.11   BDE

Immediately after a fracture, a haematoma forms at the site. A vascular pannus is associated with rheumatoid disease. Two specialised cell types are involved in fracture healing: osteoblasts lay down seams of uncalcified new bone; osteoclasts reabsorb bone and play a key role in remodelling. Immediately after a fracture, haemorrhage results in the formation of a blood clot, which is invaded by macrophages and replaced by granulation tissue. The inflammatory process extends to involve the periosteum on either side of the fracture. Bony necrosis is seen after 24–48 hours. A provisional callus of woven bone is laid down; this is then slowly reabsorbed and replaced with lamellar bone.

2.12   ACD

Myocardial blood flow is approximately 250 ml/min at rest (which represents 5% of the cardiac output) and is dependent on arterial pressure. The right coronary artery supplies a third of the blood to the left ventricular muscle. Myocardial blood flow is seen only in diastole. Pain and vasopressin (ADH) may reduce myocardial blood flow. Coronary vessels have both α- and β-adrenergic receptors. Coronary vessels generally have more α receptors and therefore vasoconstrict slightly with sympathetic stimulation.

2.13   ABDE

IPPV creates a positive intrathoracic pressure (this is normally negative) and a compression tamponade, thereby reducing venous return, cardiac output and therefore blood pressure. With a reduction in cardiac output there is reduction in liver, kidney and intestinal blood flow. The alveoli may be subjected to high inflation pressures and result in subsequent P_{CO_2} barotrauma and pneumothorax. IPPV causes an increase in intracranial pressure, as do positive end-expiratory pressure (PEEP) ventilation and obstruction of central venous drainage.

2.14   A
Cardiac index = cardiac output/body surface area. (It allows comparison of cardiac function corrected for size of the individual.) Cardiac output = stroke volume × heart rate. Systemic vascular resistance = [(mean arterial pressure – CVP)/cardiac output] × 80.

2.15   CD
Heart rate is determined by the electrical discharge of the SA node and is normally 60–80/min. The SA node spontaneously fires at 140/min and resting vagal tone reduces this to approximately 70/min. Baroreceptors in the carotid and aortic sinuses produce a reflex response to hypertension by inhibiting the SA node and decreasing the heart rate. Inspiration increases heart rate and decreases blood pressure via stretch receptors in the lung and the respiratory centre in the medulla.

2.16   BE
FRC is the volume of gas in the lung after a normal expiration. It can be calculated from the total lung capacity minus the vital capacity. FRC can be measured by the helium dilution technique or body plethysmography. FRC is often increased in diseases where there is increased airway resistance, such as emphysema, chronic bronchitis and asthma. A reduced FRC is seen in patients with reduced lung compliance, as in diffuse interstitial fibrosis.

2.17   All true
The JVP is a measure of pressure in the right atrium and usually reflects intravascular volume reasonably well. However, there are a few instances where a falsely elevated JVP may occur, as in conditions that cause or lead to right-sided cardiac failure or pulmonary hypertension.

2.18   BCD
FRC represents the volume of the lungs at the end of a normal tidal breath. It is reduced intraoperatively because of the increased activity of muscles of respiration and elevation of the diaphragm. Pain and splinting of the diaphragm occur postoperatively in abdominal surgery. With age there is loss of elastic tissue and hence the FRC rises.

2.19   CE
Dopamine at low doses has an effect on pure dopaminergic receptors; only at higher doses does it have a truly inotropic effect via β receptors. Calcium and digoxin are both inotropes. Furosemide (frusemide) and GTN may have an indirect inotropic effect if used to offload a failing ventricle, but they themselves are not inotropic. Isoprenaline is a chronotropic agent and is occasionally used in bradycardic states.

2.20   ACD
At rest, there is tonic vagal tone on the heart. This is lost after cardiac denervation and, as a result, the heart rate increases. Adenosine induces heart block, and if given in sufficient doses can cause transient asystole. Salbutamol and adrenaline have β effects on the heart and cause a tachycardia. Metronidazole has no effect on the heart rate.

2.21   DE
Angiotensin II stimulates aldosterone synthesis and secretion through the activity of a specific receptor found in the zona glomerulosa. Angiotensin II is one of the most potent endogenous vasoconstrictor agents and inhibits renin release through a negative-feedback loop. Renin stimulates the formation of angiotensin I from angiotensinogen. Angiotensin I is converted to angiotensin II in the lung by angiotensin-converting enzyme (ACE).

2.22   ABDF
Vasoconstriction is widespread and occurs on both the venous and arterial sides of the circulation. The result is increased peripheral resistance to blood flow. Changes in vascular pressures lead to an influx of extracellular water into the circulation, a phenomenon known as 'transcapillary refilling'. This leads to haemodilution. Tachycardia occurs as the blood pressure falls, which is sensed by baroreceptors in the carotid arteries and aortic arch.

2.23   AB
The CVP reflects the pressure in the right atrium and so is elevated in right-sided heart failure. The Valsalva manoeuvre raises CVP by impeding venous return to the heart. CVP is low in all types of shock, except for cardiogenic shock. CVP does not directly reflect cardiac output and, at best, is an indicator of intravascular fluid volume.

2.24   ACE
The oxygen–haemoglobin dissociation curve is sigmoid-shaped and reaches a plateau at 70–100 mmHg (PO_2). A left shift is produced by a high pH, alkalosis, a fall in PCO_2, a fall in temperature or a fall in 2,3-DPG concentration. As a result of a left shift, less oxygen is released (a higher percentage saturation for a given PO_2, leading to a fall in oxygen delivery). Anaemia produces no shift of the curve but alters the percentage oxygen saturation of the blood.

2.25   CE
Shock is inadequate tissue perfusion and inadequate delivery of oxygen and other nutrients to tissues. Of all the shock states, cardiogenic shock is unique in that cardiac output is reduced and the systemic arteriolar vessels constrict, increasing the SVR in an attempt to maintain the blood pressure. In all other forms of shock there is a primary vasodilatation of inappropriate vascular beds, causing maldistribution of blood flow. This inappropriate vasodilatation causes a fall in SVR and blood pressure. Cardiac output increases passively as a result of reduced afterload on the heart, and actively as a result of increased sympathetic drive.

2.26   ABE
Neurological complications are not uncommon following cardio-pulmonary bypass and usually manifest clinically as mild neuro-psychological deficits, such as poor short-term memory, lack of concentration and mood changes. These deficits are usually reversible and thought to result from cerebral microemboli or hypoperfusion. Fewer than 1% of patients suffer a severe stroke. Cardiopulmonary bypass causes platelet depletion and also reduces platelet activity. Acute pancreatitis occurs in 25% of open-heart procedures and may be severe in 5% of cases.

2.27   BEF
Cardiac output is decreased upon standing from a lying position as venous return to the heart is suddenly reduced. Above a certain heart rate the stroke volume falls, so reducing cardiac output. Cardiac output is increased only in the short term, when high altitude is first reached. After this initial rise, cardiac output gradually returns to normal but the haematocrit level increases to improve the blood's oxygen-carrying capacity. Other causes of increased cardiac output include arteriovenous shunts, hyperthyroidism, severe anaemia and Paget's disease.

2.40   BCD

The oxygen–haemoglobin dissociation curve is sigmoid-shaped, and a right shift is associated with a decreased affinity for oxygen. The curve shifts to the right with an increase in P_{CO_2}, temperature, 2,3-DPG and an increase in hydrogen-ion concentration (decreased pH). The curve shifts to the left with decreased P_{CO_2}, temperature, 2,3-DPG and a reduced hydrogen-ion concentration (increased pH).

2.41   ABC

PAOP can be used to exclude oedema of cardiac origin. It may be useful in cardiogenic shock to allow more accurate fluid management. PAOP may be of use in abdominal aortic aneurysm surgery. The pulmonary artery wedge pressure is elevated in cardiogenic shock. Pulmonary artery wedge pressures are not routinely measured following an MI.

2.42   ADE

The jugular venous pulsation has a double waveform. The 'a' wave corresponds to atrial contraction and ends synchronously with the carotid artery pulse. The 'c' wave occurs when the ventricles begin to contract and is caused by bulging of the atrioventricular (AV) valves backwards towards the atria. The 'v' wave is seen when the tricuspid valve is closed, just before ventricular contraction – with and just after the carotid pulse. The 'v' wave represents the gradual build-up of blood in the atria while the AV valves are closed during ventricular contraction. The absence of 'a' waves is a feature of atrial fibrillation.

2.43   CD

The total volume of CSF is approximately 150 ml. The rate of CSF production is about 550 ml/day. The composition of CSF is essentially the same as that of brain extracellular fluid. The pH of CSF is 7.33, whereas that of plasma is 7.4 due to the higher P_{CO_2} in CSF than in plasma. The protein, glucose, lactic acid, cholesterol, potassium and calcium concentrations of CSF are all lower than in plasma. However, CSF does contain more glucose than nasal mucus; so a positive glucose dipstix test of clear nasal discharge indicates a CSF leak. The lumbar CSF pressure is normally 7–18 cmH_2O.

2.28   ADE

The FRC is the residual volume plus the expiratory reserve volume and represents < 50% of the vital capacity. FRC decreases when supine and increases on standing. It also varies with height and body build. Expiratory reserve can be measured directly by spirometry, but residual volume is measured by the helium dilution technique.

2.29   BDE

The spirometer is able to measure the forced vital capacity (not the total lung capacity), the FEV_1 (forced expiratory volume in 1 second) and so the FEV_1:FVC (forced vital capacity) ratio. Residual volume is measured by helium dilution. The peak expiratory flow rate measures the amount of air expired in 1 second and extrapolates it to the volume that would be expired in 1 minute (and so can be calculated by measuring the FEV_1).

2.30   C

Pulse oximetry measures the oxygen saturation of arterial blood (not the partial pressure of oxygen). This relationship is sigmoid and not linear. Pulse oximetry does not reflect whether delivery to the tissues is adequate as this is dependent also on cardiac output and haemoglobin concentration. The adequacy of ventilation is better reflected by the P_{CO_2}. Carbon monoxide leads to the presence of carboxyhaemoglobin, which decreases the oxygen available to the tissues. Pulse oximeter readings > 95% reflect the adequacy of arterial oxygen saturation in the peripheries, nothing more. Readings can be unreliable when there is poor peripheral perfusion (in vasoconstriction, hypothermia, severe anaemia, excess ambient light, and patient movement).

2.31   CE

Finding results that are not statistically significant when the populations are actually different is known as type II error. The difference can be missed due to a combination of small sample size or high variability. Finding a statistically significant result when the populations are identical is called type I error. The Gaussian (normal) distribution plays an important role in statistical analysis. An unpaired t-test compares two groups on the assumption that the two populations are Gaussian. Paired t-tests compare two paired groups. Parametric tests are used when data from population groups follow a Gaussian distribution. Non-parametric tests are used when data from the population group does not follow a Gaussian distribution.

2.32   CE

The mean of a set of values is the same as the average. The median is the middle value of the set of values. The standard deviation (SD) is a measure of the variability of a set of values: 68% of values lie within one SD on each side of the mean, and 95% within 2 SDs of the mean. Parametric tests are used for the assessment of data that follow a Gaussian (normal) distribution, and non-parametric tests for data not following a Gaussian distribution. The outcome of a rank or score has a limited range, and an arbitrary and artificial difference between scores. Such data cannot be Gaussian in distribution.

2.33   A

Alpha-adrenoreceptor blockers will cause postural hypotension, and so decrease coronary artery perfusion. So, α stimulation will cause increased coronary artery perfusion. All β-adrenoreceptor agonists dilate the coronary vessels.

2.34   DFG

The first heart sound represents atrioventricular (AV) valve closure; the second heart sound represents aortic and pulmonary valve closure. In the cardiac cycle, the following waves/pressure changes are seen in the atria:

- The 'a' wave is caused by atrial contraction (pressure rises by 4–6 mmHg).
- The 'c' wave occurs when the ventricles begin to contract, caused by bulging of the AV valves backwards, towards the atria.
- The 'v' wave occurs towards the end of ventricular contraction, and results from the slow build-up of blood in the atria while the AV valves are closed during ventricular contraction.

2.35   ACE

Pulmonary artery occlusion (or wedge) pressure can be directly measured by Swan–Ganz catheterisation. Cardiac index and left ventricular stroke work can also be derived from these measurements using the Fick principle. FIO_2 (concentration of inspired oxygen) and end-tidal CO_2 (concentration of expired CO_2) cannot be measured by Swan–Ganz catheterisation.

2.36   ABE

Both t-tests and ANOVA (analysis of variance) are examples of parame tests and can be used to assess Gaussian (normally) distributed data. Wilcoxon and Mann–Whitney tests are non-parametric tests and are u for non-Gaussian data.

2.37   BCD

Suxamethonium is a very rapid-acting muscle relaxant and is ideal if intubation is required. Suxamethonium acts by mimicking acetylchol the neuromuscular junction but undergoes hydrolysis much more s than acetylcholine. Depolarisation is therefore prolonged, which res neuromuscular blockade. Guanethidine is an adrenergic neurob preventing the release of noradrenaline (norepinephrine) fro postganglionic adrenergic neurones. It is rarely used clinically, o resistant hypertension. Pentazocine, like fentanyl, is an opioid an Bupivacaine is a long-acting amide local anaesthetic, commonly u epidural and spinal anaesthesia. Local anaesthetics depress condu small unmyelinated fibres first and larger myelinated fibres last. It affect autonomic nerve fibres. Hexamethonium is an agent that depolarising block on the postganglionic cell body. Although it was the control of blood pressure several years ago, it is now no longe

2.38   BCE

Wound healing by secondary intention occurs when the wound not brought together. This could be due to tissue loss or wound d caused by a wound infection. The surgeon may have chosen to wound to heal by secondary intention, particularly in cases contaminated wounds. The process of wound healing by intention is much slower than primary intention, because the wound has to fill with granulation tissue and epithelialisatio occur from the wound edges.

2.39   ACE

At higher doses of adrenaline (epinephrine), α-mediated vasc reduces renal blood flow and can cause oliguria and prec renal failure. Noradrenaline (norepinephrine) is predor α agonist. Dopexamine is a potent splanchnic vasodilat afterload and improving blood flow to vital organs, including Dobutamine reduces systemic vascular resistance, decreas and ventricular filling pressures, and is of use in cardiogen cardiac failure.

2.44   DE
Calcitonin acts to oppose parathyroid hormone, and it therefore causes increased renal excretion and reduces bone resorption. Vitamin D is produced in the skin by sunlight and is ingested in the diet. It first undergoes 25-hydroxylation in the liver and then 1α-hydroxylation in the kidney to form the active 1,25-dihydroxycholecalciferol (1,25-DHCC). This last stage is under the control of PTH and phosphorus. A rise in PTH or a fall in serum phosphate increases 1,25-DHCC synthesis. Oestrogen increases calcium absorption and protects against the unopposed action of PTH.

2.45   ACD
Saliva is always hypotonic to plasma. The pH of saliva from resting glands is slightly acidic. During active secretion, however, the saliva becomes more basic, and its pH increases to nearly 8. The concentration of potassium in saliva is always much greater than its concentration in plasma. When salivary flow rates are very low, salivary potassium levels are high. The serous acinar cells have zymogen granules that contain salivary amylase – a major digestive function of saliva – which breaks down starch.

2.46   D
Blood volume is 85 ml/kg, so a 3-kg baby would have a blood volume of 255 ml. The kidneys of a neonate are not mature and therefore cannot handle large sodium loads. Heat loss is of paramount importance in neonates, and theatres should be at 25 °C to prevent excessive heat loss. Due to the immature gut, parenteral nutrition is commonly used in babies following bowel operations as they cannot cope with gastric feeds. Oral feed should be given at approximately 150 ml/kg/day in the first week.

2.47   BCDE
Prolactin secretion is controlled by the hypothalamus through the release of dopamine, which has an inhibitory effect. There are no known hypothalamic prolactin-releasing hormones, although both TRH and VIP stimulate prolactin secretion – this is not, however, of physiological importance. Prolactin secretion increases after surgery, and trauma, as part of the stress response. A physiological rise in prolactin levels is seen during pregnancy and breast-feeding. Prolactin stimulates the secretion of breast milk and reduces gonadal activity. Other common causes of hyperprolactinaemia are a prolactin-secreting tumour and drugs such as dopaminergic-receptor blockers.

2.48 AB

Insulin affects many organs and intracellular pathways. Insulin is synthesised by the β islet cells of the pancreas and is an anabolic hormone. It stimulates glucose storage but inhibits glucose production. In addition, it enhances protein synthesis and inhibits proteolysis. The uptake of glucose by the brain is independent of insulin.

2.49 ABC

The ascending and transverse colon are involved in the regulation of intraluminal fluid volume as well as sodium and water absorption. The left colon is the site for final modulation of intraluminal contents before evacuation. More than 90% of short-chain fatty acids are taken up by colonic mucosal cells. Chloride absorption occurs by a passive energy-independent mechanism, being absorbed together with sodium. Bicarbonate is secreted by the colon, by an energy-requiring process. Bile salts are absorbed in the terminal ileum.

2.50 BE

The terminal ileum is the primary site for absorption of the fat-soluble vitamins B_{12} and K. In addition, bile salts are predominantly absorbed here. Calcium and folic acid are mainly absorbed in the jejunum.

2.51 ACD

One of the functions of the spleen is the sequestration and phagocytosis of old or abnormal red cells. Therefore, in a postsplenectomy patient, red-cell inclusion bodies may be present, producing target cells, Howell–Jolly bodies and sideroblasts. Punctate basophilia is seen in patients with lead poisoning, thalassaemia, and haemolytic anaemia due to pyrimidine-5-nucleotidase deficiency. Rouleaux formation is the tendency for red cells to stack up like a pile of coins. The amount of rouleaux formation is determined by the concentration of protein in the plasma.

2.52   AB
The pancreas is an essential endocrine organ that produces insulin, glucagon and other hormones. Pancreatic secretion is alkaline, which maintains the correct pH levels for enzyme action and function. The exocrine function of the pancreas is to produce enzymes for normal digestion. Inactive precursors of these enzymes are secreted in pancreatic juice and cleaved to form trypsin and chymotrypsin, as well as carboxypeptidases, lipase, co-lipase and amylase. Secretion of pancreatic juice is primarily under the control of two hormones – secretin and cholecystokinin (CCK) – secreted by the duodenum. The rate of pancreatic secretion is typically 150 ml/h and therefore approximately 3500 ml/day.

2.53   CE
Neural and hormonal signals control pancreatic exocrine secretion. The main trigger is the presence of acid and products of digestion in the duodenum, not the presence of triglycerides. Lipase is secreted by glands near the base of the tongue (responsible for up to 30% of triglyceride digestion), and the remainder is digested by pancreatic lipase – which requires a cofactor (co-lipase) to become active. The products of triglyceride breakdown are free fatty acids and 2-monoglycerides.

2.54   ACD
Following a meal, cholecystokinin is secreted by the duodenum and stimulates contraction of the gallbladder and relaxation of the sphincter of Oddi, so allowing bile to enter the duodenum. Bile salts are involved in the absorption of fat through the formation of micelles. Bile salts are absorbed in the terminal ileum and transported back to the liver. This forms part of the enterohepatic circulation and prevents excessive loss of bile salts. Bile salts have a stimulating action on the gut, increasing mobility and thereby decreasing bowel transit times. Failure to absorb bile salts will cause diarrhoea.

2.55   ABCDFG
Chronic alcohol abuse may cause a Wernicke's encephalopathy (a reversible condition) and Korsakoff's syndrome (irreversible). Signs and symptoms of cerebellar ataxia are common in chronic alcoholism. Other effects of chronic alcohol ingestion include generalised marrow depression, with lymphopenia and immunosuppression. Macrocytosis is generally due to decreased folate levels, caused by chronic alcohol abuse. Sydenham's chorea is associated with rheumatic fever.

2.56 ABD
The colon absorbs up to 5 litres of water a day. The colonic mucosa actively absorbs sodium and chloride ions, whereas bicarbonate accumulates on the mucosal side. Chloride ions are actively absorbed against a large concentration gradient. Chloride and bicarbonate exchange has been estimated to provide 25% of total absorption in the colon. Short-chain fatty acids are produced by anaerobic fermentation of undigested carbohydrates by colonic bacteria.

2.57 ADE
Average-sized term infants require 150 ml/kg of formula feed per day. This will provide about 100 calories (419 J)/kg per day (the basic nutritional requirement). When a newborn infant undergoes surgery and requires intravenous fluids, he or she will require 100 ml of water/kg/day as well as 3 mmol sodium and 2 mmol potassium/kg/day. An infant undergoing surgery is under stress, and is at risk of hypoglycaemia. Therefore, a solution of 10% dextrose with 0.9% saline, to which is added 10 ml of potassium per 500 ml, will meet the infant's basic maintenance needs. Around 95% of term infants should pass meconium within the first 24 hours. Failure to do so might indicate a diagnosis of Hirschsprung's disease.

2.58 CD
All the body's potassium is potentially exchangeable, most of it being intracellular (89.6%). Hence, the plasma level of potassium is not a good indicator of total body potassium. In contrast, only 9% of sodium is intracellular. The extracellular potassium (% of total body level) is found in bone (7.6%), connective tissue and cartilage (0.4%), plasma (0.4%), interstitial fluid (1%) and transcellular locations (1%). There is a correlation between potassium and hydrogen ions, the two rising and falling together. Aldosterone is a steroid hormone secreted by the zona glomerulosa in the adrenal gland. It causes increased reabsorption of sodium from urine, sweat, saliva and gastric juice. In the kidney, aldosterone acts on the epithelium of the distal convoluted tubule and collecting ducts to increase sodium retention and potassium loss.

2.59   D

The plasma concentration of potassium is 4–5 mmol/l. The CSF contains 2.9 mmol/l of potassium, saliva 6–8 mmol/l, sweat 5 mmol/l gastric juice 10 mmol/l and ileostomy fluid 10 mmol/l. The major electrolytes in saliva are sodium, potassium, chloride and bicarbonate. Their concentrations are similar to those found in plasma, although a richer, potassium-containing fluid may result in the primary secretion being hypertonic. This is all dependent on saliva flows (low saliva flow, high potassium).

2.60   ABCD

Acute tubular necrosis would elevate plasma potassium. Aldosterone lowers serum potassium by increasing loss in the distal convoluted tubule and collecting ducts of the kidney. The extracellular fluid compartment contains potassium, and depletion would lead to hypokalaemia. Diarrhoea fluid contains between 35–60 mmol/l of potassium, hence hypokalaemia can occur readily. A fall in plasma potassium is associated with a rise in pH, hence metabolic alkalosis.

2.61   ABE

The most common biochemical abnormality in pyloric stenosis is a hypochloraemic alkalosis. This leads to a compensatory rise in arterial P_{CO_2}. Due to dehydration, urea levels will increase. Hypokalaemia is a feature of prolonged vomiting in pyloric stenosis, as gastric juice is rich in potassium (10 mmol/l).

2.62   ABD

The intracellular component of body water accounts for about 40% of body weight, and the extracellular component 20%. In health, the intracellular and extracellular pH are maintained at very constant levels: pH 7.40 ± 0.05. Intracellular fluid has higher concentrations of potassium, phosphate, protein and magnesium compared with extracellular fluid; but lower sodium, chloride and bicarbonate levels.

2.63   DE

Plasma volume is measured by using dyes (such as Evans blue) that become bound to plasma·protein. Plasma volume can also be indirectly measured by injecting serum albumin labelled with radioactive iodine. Radioactive inulin can be used to measure extracellular fluid volume.

2.64 ABD

At rest, the kidney receives 25% of the cardiac output, approx 1.2 litres of blood/minute. Renal plasma flow can be measured by infusing PAH and determining its urine and plasma concentrations. PAH is filtered by the glomeruli and secreted by the renal tubular cells, so its excretion ratio is high. The effective renal plasma flow is equivalent to the urine clearance of PAH. Blood flow in the renal cortex is much higher than in the medulla. The factors affecting renal blood flow include: blood volume (hypovolaemia reduces renal blood flow) and catecholamines (constrict renal vessels so reducing flow). ADH causes water retention, the effect of which is to increase renal blood flow.

2.65 ACD

The descending loop of Henle is permeable to water but the ascending loop is impermeable. Sodium, potassium and chloride are co-transported out of the thick segment of the ascending limb. Therefore, a gradient exists whereby the fluid in the descending loop of Henle becomes hypertonic as water moves into the hypertonic interstitium (sodium level increases as the descending limb travels downwards). In the ascending limb, the fluid in the tubules becomes more dilute and is hypotonic to plasma because of movement of sodium and chloride out of the tubular lumen. This forms the mechanism of the counter-current multiplier.

2.66 ABC

Renin secretion is increased by stimuli that decrease ECF volume and blood pressure or increase sympathetic output. So, the stimuli that increase renin secretion include: sodium depletion, cardiac failure, dehydration, constriction of the renal artery, hypotension, haemorrhage and an upright posture. Renin is responsible for the conversion of angiotensinogen to angiotensin I. Angiotensin-converting enzyme is responsible for the conversion of angiotensin I to angiotensin II (predominantly in the lungs). Renin is produced by the juxtaglomerular cells, which, together with the macula densa and lacis cells, constitute the juxtaglomerular apparatus.

2.67   BCD

Dehydration leads to splanchnic and visceral vasoconstriction, so renal blood flow falls. This causes a drop in urine output and a minimum obligatory urine output of 500 ml/24 h may result. The secretion of antidiuretic hormone (ADH) leading to increased water reabsorption is another mechanism by which this occurs. The loops of Henle of the juxtamedullary nephrons dip deeply into the medullary pyramids before draining into the distal convoluted tubules in the cortex. There is a graded increase in the osmolality at the tips of the papillae (around 1200 mOsm/l approximately equal to four times that of plasma).

2.68   ABD

The mechanisms of oxygen release from blood to the peripheral tissues are determined by factors shifting the oxygen–haemoglobin dissociation curve. Hence, a low pH state, increase in temperature, increase in PCO_2 and an increase in 2,3-DPG all facilitate the delivery of oxygen to the tissues, by raising the PO_2 at which O_2 is released in the peripheral capillaries (shift of the curve to the right).

2.69   AD

In arterial blood, 89.4% of the CO_2 is in the form of HCO_3^-. Only 5.3% is in carbamino compounds and 5.3% is dissolved in plasma. CO_2 is about 20 times more soluble than O_2 in simple solutions at equal partial pressure. CO_2 readily diffuses into red blood cells and is rapidly hydrated to H_2CO_3 in the presence of carbonic anhydrase. The H_2CO_3 dissociates into H^+ and HCO_3^-, and the H^+ is buffered mainly by haemoglobin, while the HCO_3^- enters the plasma.

2.70   All true

Lung compliance can be defined as the change in lung volume per unit change in airway pressure. It is normally measured in the steepest part of the relaxation pressure curve (normal value 0.2 l/cmH$_2$O). The surface tension of the film of fluid that lines the alveoli is an important factor affecting lung compliance. Any injury to the lung can reduce compliance. A low lung compliance equates to having a 'stiffer' lung.

2.71   BCDE

Chemoreceptors found in the carotid and aortic bodies are sensitive to changes in the chemistry of blood, resulting in stimulation of the respiratory centre. So, an increase in respiratory rate causes a respiratory alkalosis. Arterial blood pressure would also rise indirectly, increasing blood flow to the brain.

2.72   ABCE

Pulmonary ventilation is stimulated by acidosis, hypercapnia and hypoxia, mediated via respiratory chemoreceptors in the carotid and aortic bodies and medulla of the brain. The respiratory centre is not located in the cerebellum, but in the medulla and pons.

2.73   AE

A tracheostomy will decrease the anatomical dead space but not the physiological dead space. Anatomical dead space is the respiratory system volume exclusive of the alveoli. Physiological dead space is the volume of gas not equilibrating with blood, or wasted ventilation. In normal healthy individuals, the two dead spaces are identical. Airway resistance and lung compliance would also be improved by tracheostomy and this is one of the advantages of such a procedure. A tracheostomy would have no effect on the residual lung volume or vital capacity.

2.74   ABE

Major abdominal surgery causes pain resulting in reduced tidal volumes. Decreased minute ventilatory volume would also be a feature. In uncomplicated major abdominal surgery, lung compliance is unaffected. However, if the patient were to develop adult respiratory disease syndrome (ARDS) then lung compliance would fall.

2.75   DE

Baroreceptors are stretch receptors found in the adventitia of the blood vessels and wall of the heart. The arterial baroreceptors are located in the carotid sinus and aortic arch. When the arterial blood pressure drops, the arterial wall is subjected to less stretch, and the sensory nerves coming from the carotid sinus (sinus nerve) and from the aortic arch (depressor nerve) become less active and send fewer impulses. Upon receiving fewer impulses from the baroreceptors, the cardiovascular centres respond by exciting the sympathetic and inhibiting the parasympathetic nervous systems. This leads to an increase in heart rate and stroke volume, and generalised constriction of arterioles (not brain or heart) and veins. On the venous side, receptors are found in the wall of the left and right atria, at the entrances of the inferior vena cava and superior vena cava and in the pulmonary circulation.

2.76   CD
The carotid body (like the aortic body) is a peripheral chemoreceptor. It is stimulated by a drop in arterial Po_2 or a rise in arterial Pco_2. This results in a compensatory increase in ventilation. The blood flow in the carotid body is enormous: 2000 ml/100 g tissue per minute. The central chemoreceptors in the medulla on the ventral surface of the brainstem monitor hydrogen ion concentration of cerebrospinal fluid. Carbon dioxide readily passes through the blood–brain barrier and parallels the hydrogen ion concentration in the interstitial fluid of the brain.

2.77   BCDE
During vigorous exercise the CVP would remain unchanged or may fall with dehydration. In exercise, the stroke volume increases, with a decrease in end-systolic volume. With the increase in heart rate, the end-diastolic volume may also increase slightly as less time is spent by the heart in diastole.

2.78   ACE
Cerebral blood flow is affected by arterial blood pressure, venous blood pressure, intracranial pressure, viscosity of the blood and the vascular resistance of the cerebral arterioles. The calibre of the arterioles are controlled by local vasodilator metabolites such as Pco_2, angiotensin II and autoregulatory mechanisms. Raised intracranial pressure would reduce cerebral blood flow. Noradrenaline would increase arterial blood pressure and therefore cerebral blood flow.

2.79   ABDE
Blood flow in exercising muscle is mainly influenced by local mechanisms. Factors increasing blood flow in muscle include: fall in tissue Po_2, rise in tissue Pco_2, accumulation of potassium and vasodilator metabolites (such as bradykinin). An increase in temperature would also dilate vessels, increasing the cross-sectional area of the vascular bed and thereby reducing blood flow velocity. Blood flow in muscle doubles after sympathectomy. The parasympathetic nervous system has no known effects on muscle blood flow.

2.80   CD
By definition in hypovolaemic shock, there is a fall in cardiac output with a lowering of the CVP. The body's response to this is splanchnic vasoconstriction with reduced blood flow to the skin and viscera. Cerebral perfusion will be maintained initially by autoregulatory mechanisms but once these are exceeded, cerebral blood flow will also drop.

2.81 BE

Secretin is secreted by S cells found in the proximal small bowel. It increases the secretion of bicarbonate by the duct cells of the pancreas (causes secretion of a watery, alkaline pancreatic juice) and biliary tract, augments the action of cholecystokinin, decreases gastric acid secretion and causes pyloric sphincter contraction. The secretion of secretin is increased by acid from the duodenum and by products of protein digestion.

2.82 BE

Glycerol, monoglycerides and long-chain fatty acids move into mucosal cells where they are re-esterified into triglycerides, which are then packaged along with cholesterol into large lipoprotein particles (chylomicrons). These are then transported out of the cell into the lacteals. Short-chain fatty acids pass directly through the cells into the blood. Cholesterol is readily absorbed from the small intestine if bile, fatty acids and pancreatic juice are present. Fat absorption is greatest in the upper parts of the small intestine, but significant amounts are absorbed in the ileum.

2.83 AB

The colon has a large absorptive capacity. Sodium is actively transported out of the colon along with water. Chloride ions are also absorbed. Potassium and bicarbonate are normally secreted into the colon. Bile salts are absorbed in the terminal ileum as part of the enterohepatic circulation. Amino acid absorption occurs rapidly in the duodenum and jejunum, but it is slow in the ileum.

2.84 ABE

Iron absorption is dependent on iron being in the reduced ferrous state (Fe^{2+}) and acid from the stomach and duodenum is predominantly responsible for this. Intrinsic factor is a glycoprotein produced by the stomach and is a cofactor required for the absorption of vitamin B_{12} (cyanocobalamin). Cyanocobalamin becomes firmly bound to intrinsic factor in the small intestine. This complex then becomes bound to specific receptors in the terminal ileum, and cyanocobalamin is transferred across the intestinal epithelium. Trypsin is required for this process to be efficient.

2.85 A

Sweating is a cholinergic impulse response. Adrenaline only has a minimal effect on sweating, causing slight localised secretion. Tachycardia and paroxysmal hypertension are features of high circulating levels of adrenaline. Hepatic glucose output is also seen, giving rise to hyperglycaemia and glycosuria.

2.86   ACD

Adrenaline exerts its effects by stimulation of β_1 and β_2 receptors: it increases the force (inotropic) and rate (chronotropic) of contraction of the heart; β_1 effects – adrenaline dilates blood vessels in skeletal muscle and liver; β_2 effects – splanchnic vasoconstriction occurs with administration of adrenaline through its α effect (small). Decreased bowel motility is seen with adrenaline, mediated through α and β_2 effects. Bronchodilatation is produced through relaxation of the bronchial muscle (β_2 effect).

2.87   ABCE

A prolonged elevation of plasma cortisol would produce a clinical picture of Cushing's syndrome. Protein depletion is a feature as a result of excess protein catabolism. The amino acids liberated from the catabolism of proteins are converted into glucose in the liver. A resultant hyperglycaemia is seen, and this may precipitate diabetes mellitus. Cortisol can exert a significant mineralocorticoid action, so causing sodium retention and potassium loss. Excess cortisol also has the effect of decreasing bone formation and increasing bone resorption, leading to osteoporosis and loss of bone mass.

2.88   ABE

The anterior pituitary gland secretes six hormones: thyroid-stimulating hormone (TSH, thyrotropin), growth hormone, adrenocorticotropic hormone (ACTH), luteinising hormone (LH), follicle-stimulating hormone (FSH) and prolactin. The posterior pituitary secretes oxytocin and vasopressin. Calcitonin is produced by the parafollicular C cells of the thyroid. Calcitonin lowers the circulating calcium and phosphate, although the exact physiological role of calcitonin is unknown. Aldosterone is secreted from the zona glomerulosa of the adrenal gland.

2.89   ABCD

Proprioceptive information is conveyed in the dorsal white columns of the spinal cord. Much of this information goes to the cerebellum but some is also conveyed to the cortex. The sensory afferents for cold (Aδ and C fibres) and warm (C fibres) relay information to the postcentral gyrus via the lateral spinothalamic tract and the thalamic radiation. Nociceptive afferents end in the spinal cord and brainstem, thalamus, postcentral gyrus and peri-aqueductal grey matter.

2.90   ABDE

In surgery, sodium depletion is synonymous with extracellular fluid loss: gastrointestinal losses (vomiting, diarrhoea, fistula). Sodium is never lost without water and so hence in severe sodium depletion, the patient will be hypovolaemic. This subsequently stimulates the body's homeostatic mechanisms.

2.91   ABC

The first part of the distal convoluted tubule is effectively an extension of the thick segment of the loop of Henle, and is therefore relatively impermeable to water. The reabsorption of sodium in this segment is regulated by aldosterone. Aldosterone also has the effect of increasing the secretion of potassium and hydrogen ions into the tubular lumen. Approximately 5% of the filtered water is removed in this segment of the kidney. ADH acts predominantly on the collecting ducts to increase their permeability to water, so leading to water retention.

2.92   ABC

Humans can tolerate body temperatures of 21–24 °C without permanent ill effects. Hypothermia is often used in cardiac surgery. Total circulatory arrest occurs at temperatures below 19 °C. The oxygen needs of the tissues are greatly reduced at low temperatures. Hypothermia causes a shift of the oxygen dissociation curve to the left, so increasing the oxygen content of blood at a given tension. Blood viscosity increases with a fall in body temperature.

2.93   AB

Glucose is the major direct source of energy for the brain under normal conditions. Glucose enters the brain via a glucose transporter system. In prolonged starvation, pregnancy and in the newborn, the brain develops the capacity to use ketone bodies for energy. Ketone bodies are formed from the condensation of acetyl CoA following the degredation of fatty acids in the liver.

2.94   B
Glycogen, the storage form of glucose, is present in most body tissues but mainly in the liver and skeletal muscle. Insulin is the main substance that stimulates glycogen formation. Glucagon stimulates glycogenolysis by increasing intracellular cAMP levels. Adrenaline stimulates glycogenolysis by increasing intracellular calcium levels. The glycogen content of a normal liver is 70–100 g, which is sufficient to maintain plasma glucose for only 8 hours. Cortisol limits the utilisation of glucose but in the long term elevates plasma glucose concentrations.

2.95   ABC
Hypomagnesaemia should be suspected in patients with malnutrition, excess alcohol ingestion, prolonged diuretic treatment and chronic mineralocorticoid excess. Both alcohol and diuretics increase magnesium excretion. Hypomagnesaemia can produce hypocalcaemia and contribute to the persistence of hypokalaemia (renal potassium wasting). The main site of magnesium absorption is the duodenum. Mild magnesium deficiency may be treated with oral supplements but in severe cases slow intravenous infusion is required.

2.96   B
Metabolic rate is affected by a number of factors including muscular exertion (most important), ingestion of food, sex, age, height, weight, surface area, body temperature, environmental temperature, emotional state, circulating levels of thyroid hormones, adrenaline and noradrenaline.

2.97   BCD
The body responds to any form of injury (including surgery) with local and systemic responses that attempt to contain and heal the tissue damage, and also to protect the body while it is injured. The systemic response, produced by many different mediators (sympathetic nervous system, acute phase response, endocrine response and vascular endothelial cell system response), increases the metabolic rate, mobilises carbohydrate, protein and fat stores, conserves salt and water, stimulates immunological and coagulation systems, and diverts blood preferentially to vital organs. Blood is redistributed from the viscera and skin to the heart, brain and skeletal muscles, and there is an increase in heart rate and contractility. In the ebb phase after injury, plasma insulin concentration falls because catecholamines and cortisol make the β islet cells of the pancreas less sensitive to glucose. Glucagon also inhibits insulin release and cortisol reduces the peripheral action of insulin: less carbohydrate is transported into cells and blood sugar rises.

Arginine vasopressin acts on the distal tubules and collecting ducts in the kidney and leads to increased reabsorption of solute-free water; it causes peripheral vasoconstriction, especially in the splanchnic bed, and it also stimulates hepatic glycogenolysis and gluconeogenesis. In addition, glucagon secretion increases after injury, further stimulating hepatic glycogenolysis and gluconeogenesis. Adrenocorticotrophic hormone (ACTH) stimulates aldosterone secretion (in addition to glucocorticoids), which causes increased reabsorption of sodium and secretion of potassium (and hydrogen ions) in the distal convoluted tubules and collecting ducts, leading to metabolic alkalosis as well as a reduction in the urine volume. In more severe injuries, however, a metabolic acidosis is common, owing to poor tissue perfusion and anaerobic metabolism. Serum albumin falls after trauma because production by the liver decreases and loss into damaged tissue increases due to the action of cytokines and prostaglandins on vessel permeability. The accompanying fluid shift out of the intravascular compartment contributes to dysfunction in various organs.

2.98   C
Gangrene implies death with putrefaction of macroscopic portions of the tissue. A gangrenous part lacks arterial pulsation, venous return, sensation, warmth and function. Dry gangrene occurs when the tissues are desiccated by gradual slowing of the bloodstream; it is typically the result of atherosclerosis. Moist gangrene occurs when venous as well as arterial obstruction is present, when the artery is suddenly occluded, as by a ligature or embolus, and in diabetes. In moist gangrene, infection and putrefaction are more severe, the affected part becomes swollen and discoloured, and the epidermis may be raised in blebs. Diabetic gangrene is due to three factors: trophic changes resulting from peripheral neuritis; atheroma of the small arteries resulting in ischaemia; and excess sugar lowering the resistance to infection. Diabetic gangrene of the toes can occur in the presence of palpable peripheral pulses (absence implies associated major arterial disease).

Clostridium perfringens, widely found in nature, particularly soil and faeces, is the cause of gas gangrene in about 80% of cases. Wound infections are associated with severe local wound pain and crepitus; gas in the tissues may be noted on plain radiographs. Synergistic spreading gangrene (synonyms: necrotising fasciitis; Meleney's gangrene for abdominal wall infections; and Fournier's gangrene for scrotal infections) is usually caused by a mixed pattern of organisms – coliforms, staphylococci, *Bacteroides* spp., anaerobic streptococci, and peptostreptococci. The extent of subdermal spread of gangrene is always much more extensive than at first apparent. Surgical debridement, wide excision and laying open of the affected tissue, combined with broad-spectrum antibiotic therapy and aggressive circulatory support, may be necessary to save life; skin grafting, after resolution of acute symptoms, may be needed to cover the large, excised areas. Meleney's gangrene still carries a mortality of 30%.

2.99   DE

Although shearing injuries to the scalp can result in severe blood loss and external haematoma, they do not cause a raised intracranial pressure (ICP). Both extradural and subdural haematomas, and any condition leading to cerebral oedema or cerebral engorgement could lead to a rise in ICP. Likewise, obstruction to the cerebrospinal fluid (CSF) pathway could lead to a raised ICP, although this is uncommon after head injuries. In the early stages of head injury, there is a non-linear relationship between an expanding haematoma and elevation of ICP – a haematoma may expand without any significant rise in pressure. Once this early compliance is lost, the pressure will rise rapidly. This severely jeopardises cerebral perfusion: cerebral perfusion pressure (CPP) is equal to mean arterial blood pressure minus ICP (normal CPP is approximately 70 mmHg and the normal ICP in adults is 10–15 mmHg). Therefore, any rise in ICP will cause a corresponding fall in CPP.

As ICP rises, CSF is driven out of the intracranial compartment – the first stage of compensation. This follows the Monro–Kellie hypothesis which states that: The sum of intracranial volumes of blood, brain, CSF and other components is constant, and that an increase in any one of these must be offset by a corresponding decrease in another, or else ICP will rise.' With continuing rise in ICP, brain shifts occur within the cranial cavity. The most important of these brain shifts is uncal transtentorial herniation or 'coning'. This causes impairment of conscious level, development of an ipsilateral fixed dilated pupil (due to IIIrd nerve compression), hemiparesis of the contralateral side (due to compression of the cerebral peduncle), and later cardiovascular and respiratory abnormalities (Cheyne–Stokes breathing) due to brainstem compression. The agonal event is often accompanied by hypertension and bradycardia – Cushing's reflex. Frank papilloedema may be seen at this stage.

2.100   ABC

Vasoconstriction, in combination with clot formation and platelet aggregation, occurs in response to initial injury. Once aggregated, the platelets degranulate and release mediators such as adenosine diphosphate (ADP), which further expedites coagulation, plus important growth factors and chemotactic factors. These factors attract inflammatory leucocytes such as neutrophils, which help to phagocytose bacteria and other foreign bodies present within the wound. Neutrophil infiltration usually ceases within a few days, and the invading neutrophils become entrapped within the wound clot and desiccated tissue. They are also phagocytosed by tissue macrophages. In the later stages of healing, other chemoattractants, such as fragments of collagen, elastin and fibronectin, attract monocytes (macrophages are a phenotypic variation of monocytes) into the wound. They promote phagocytosis, continue debriding dead tissue by releasing enzymes, such as collagenase, and several growth factors, and also help to recruit fibroblasts, keratinocytes and endothelial cells to repair the damaged tissues. So, macrophages play a pivotal role in the transition between inflammation and repair.

The levels of various proteases, such as matrix metalloproteinases, serine proteases, and neutrophil elastase are elevated in chronic wounds. These proteases degrade vital elements of the extracellular matrix (ECM) and certain growth factors, so predisposing to chronic wounds. Hypertrophic scars and keloids are the result of aberrations in the normal progression of healing, leading to excessive ECM deposition and subsequent over- or unregulated scarring. Hypertrophic scars are confined to the borders of the original wound, but keloids extend beyond the original wound and invade surrounding tissues. Keloids are more common in wounds that cross tension lines and in areas such as the ear lobe and presternal and deltoid regions. While hypertrophic scars generally begin to develop in the weeks after injury, keloids can develop up to 1 year later.

2.101   ABC

Unconjugated bilirubin is the main breakdown product of the haem moiety of haemoglobin and is derived mostly from effete erythrocytes. Unconjugated bilirubin is insoluble in water and is transported bound to albumin in the plasma. Unconjugated bilirubin is transported across the hepatocyte membrane by a carrier protein, where it is bound to glutathione transferases, enters the endoplasmic reticulum, and is conjugated to bilirubin monoglucuronide and bilirubin diglucuronide, both of which are water-soluble. Unconjugated hyperbilirubinaemia is caused by overproduction of bilirubin, usually as a result of haemolytic disease such as spherocytosis, thalassaemia and sickle cell disease. In such disorders, the liver is presented with an excessive load of bilirubin which is unconjugated and therefore absent from the urine. However, a healthy liver attempts to conjugate the majority of the bilirubin presented to it and so the faecal stercobilinogen and urinary urobilinogen levels are raised. (Gut bacteria cause conjugated bilirubin to form urobilinogen, of which 20% is excreted in urine and 80% is excreted in stools; urobilinogen on oxidation forms urobilin, which is colourless.)

Post-hepatic jaundice (owing to bile duct obstruction, strictures, and pancreatic, bile duct and ampullary malignancies) causes a conjugated hyperbilirubinaemia with bilirubin in the urine, causing dark urine; bilirubin is absent in the stools, leading to pale stools. Pruritis is an important feature of both hepatic and post-hepatic cholestasis. Itching, which is related to bile salt deposition within the skin, is most severe on the extremities and worse in warm weather. When jaundice is caused by a stone in the common bile duct (CBD), dilatation of the gallbladder is rare, but when the duct is obstructed in some other way (such as carcinoma of the ampulla, pancreas or bile duct) dilatation is common (Courvoisier's law). This is because stones in the CBD lead to fibrosis and atrophy of the gallbladder.

2.102   BDE

Bacterial flexor tenosynovitis should be distinguished from stenosing tenosynovitis ('trigger' finger) of the digital flexor tendons. Stenosing tenosynovitis mostly affects the thumb or ring finger but can involve any digit. Bacterial flexor tenosynovitis, on the other hand, results from penetrating wounds to the hand and the majority are due to *Staphylococcus aureus* infection. Any digit can be affected depending on the site of injury. Infections of the finger flexor tendons are serious, with the potential for substantial permanent functional impairment. Finger movements are severely restricted and the four cardinal signs of tendon sheath infection are: partially flexed posture of the finger; fusiform swelling of the finger; tenderness along the entire flexor tendon sheath; and severe pain from passive extension of the finger. The tenosynovitis can rapidly destroy the synovial gliding surfaces and result in healing with restrictive adhesions. A fulminating infection can lead to tendon necrosis.

Early tenosynovitis can be treated with intravenous antibiotics, elevation and splinting. However, if no definite signs of improvement are seen after 24 hours, surgical exploration or drainage must be considered since the consequences of a fulminating flexor tenosynovitis are so severe and permanent. Initial drainage should be with a limited proximal incision in the distal palm over the tendon sheath, through which a small catheter can be introduced. A small distal incision for outflow is then made to create a through-and-through irrigation system with minimal surgical damage. For the vast majority of cases these measures, along with antibiotics and supportive care will bring the situation promptly under control. In severe cases, however, radical drainage by opening the whole finger through a mid-axial incision and opening the sheath while carefully preserving the pulleys may be required.

2.103   AC

Approximately 1 litre of saliva is produced per day. The rate of secretion increases with nausea. Saliva produced by the submandibular and sublingual glands is serous and mucous; parotid secretion is mainly mucous. Owing to active transport against a concentration gradient, saliva contains a higher concentration of potassium and a lower concentration of sodium compared to plasma. Consequently, if a large volume is lost hypokalaemia may result. Although secretion rates are reduced during sleep, secretion does not stop completely.

2.104 D

Iodine is actively transported into the thyroid gland against a concentration gradient; normal iodine concentration in the thyroid is 30 times greater than that in blood. Thyroid hormone secreted into the blood consists of predominantly T4 and T3 in a ratio of 93%:7%. However, approximately 50% of T4 produced becomes deiodinated to T3 within a few days of secretion. Both T3 and T4 are mainly bound to thyroglobulin, which is synthesised in the liver. T4 has a half-life of approximately 15 days, with some activity persisting for up to 6 weeks.

2.105 BD

Glucose will not diffuse through a cell membrane against a concentration gradient. Insulin facilitates the diffusion of glucose across many cell membranes including cardiac muscle cells, skeletal muscle cells, some smooth muscle cells and adipose tissue cells. Insulin does not affect transport of glucose into brain cells, renal tubular epithelium or across intestinal mucosa.

2.106 AC

Thyroxine has wide-ranging effects on metabolism. This hormone increases oxygen consumption in every tissue in the body and stimulates protein synthesis. Thyroxine affects both the synthesis and degradation of lipids, the net effect being a decrease in lipid stores. By influencing the mechanisms by which cholesterol is eliminated from the body, thyroxine decreases plasma cholesterol levels. Owing to its stimulatory effect on metabolic processes, thyroxine will also have the effect of increasing the demand for coenzymes and vitamins.

2.107 BC

CSF is formed mainly by the choroid plexus by an active secretory process. It circulates in the subarachnoid space and is absorbed into the circulation by the arachnoid villi. CSF glucose and protein levels are both much lower than those of plasma. Changes in these concentrations are helpful in detecting pathological processes such as tumour or infection, where the blood–brain barrier is breached.

2.108   AD

The primary effects of aldosterone on the renal system are to increase reabsorption of sodium and increase secretion of potassium and hydrogen ions. Aldosterone acts by increasing the number and activity of the active transport systems in the distal renal tubule to sodium and potassium. Owing to the enhanced reabsorption of sodium, water reabsorption is also increased. Aldosterone increases excretion of both ammonium and magnesium.

2.109   ABE

Macrophages are part of the mononuclear phagocytic system and are derived from bone marrow haemopoietic cells. Macrophages are well-known phagocytic cells. The function of macrophages includes antimicrobial defence against intracellular organisms such as *Mycobacteria, Listeria* and *Histoplasma* spp. Macrophages also play a vital role in several aspects of the immune response. They take up antigen and degrade it to short polypeptides that can be expressed on their surface. Furthermore, the macrophages play a role in delayed-type hypersensitivity reactions, and also have anti-tumour activity. In addition, they produce various colony-stimulating factors, which promote the growth and development of different white blood cells, and a number of factors that act on other cells (monokines), such as interleukin-1 (IL-1), which stimulates helper T cells. Indirectly, macrophages also promote the production of more erythrocytes, since they have a greater affinity for the iron transport compound, transferrin. Once transferrin has been converted to ferritin by phagocytes, this storage form of iron is delivered to the bone marrow where it speeds up the production of haemoglobin, which in turn shortens the maturation time of new red blood cells. Macrophages are involved in granulomatous and chronic inflammation, whereby macrophages and monocytes differentiate into epithelioid cells. Giant cells are formed by fusion of macrophages in response to exogenous insoluble material (such as talc and silica) and in reaction to endogenous insoluble material, such as keratin, fat and cholesterol, and certain organisms such as those causing tuberculosis and syphilis.

2.110   ACE

General host factors predisposing to wound infection include hypoxia, jaundice, anaemia, increasing age, obesity, uraemia, malnutrition, diabetes mellitus, hypovolaemic shock, corticosteroids and immuno-suppressants.

2.111 BE

Rising intracranial pressure presents with headache, drowsiness, vomiting and seizures and there is often a history of trauma. Signs include listlessness, irritability, drowsiness, falling pulse, rising blood pressure, coma, irregular breathing (respiratory depression from compression of the medulla) and, later, papilloedema. Lumbar puncture is contraindicated in raised intracranial pressure.

2.112 ACD

The inflammatory response is dependent on the extent of tissue injury. Inflammation is characterised by increased blood flow to the affected area, increased vascular permeability, chemotaxis of inflammatory cells and release of numerous preformed mediators such as histamine, prostaglandins, kinins and complement proteins.

2.113 ADE

Non-cycling ('resting') cells are said to be in the G0 phase of the cell cycle. RNA and protein synthesis occur during the first growth phase, G1. Duplication (replication) of cellular DNA occurs during the S phase, which is followed by a second growth phase (G2). This precedes mitosis (M). The duration of the cell cycle varies from 20 to 100 hours; (20–24 hours in rapidly growing cells). The rate of tumour growth decreases exponentially with time (Gompertzian pattern), so the growth fraction of small tumours is greater than that of larger ones. Cytotoxic drugs usually act on cycling cells and can be phase- or non-phase-specific.

2.114 AB

At normal systemic blood pressure the renal vascular resistance adjusts the pressure in the renal arterioles so that renal blood flow remains fairly constant (autoregulation). In hypertensive patients there is a shift of autoregulation, so that they have a slightly reduced renal blood flow for a given blood pressure. Blood flow in the cortex is much higher than in the medulla. Autoregulation is impaired in shock, sepsis and low cardiac output states.

2.115   AE

The gastrointestinal tract is selectively impaired in patients who are in shock. It is one of the first organs to be affected and one of the last to be restored by resuscitation. Measurement of stomach perfusion can be estimated on the basis of the intramural pH. It is measured by tonometry: a catheter is filled with saline and allowed to equilibrate with the luminal P_{CO_2}, which is assumed to be the same as the P_{CO_2} of the superficial mucosa. Determination of the arterial bicarbonate concentration will allow calculation of the intramural pH using the Henderson–Hasselbalch equation. This measurement reflects splanchnic tissue oxygenation and is an indirect and early means of estimating global tissue oxygenation.

2.116   BDE

Nitric oxide (NO), previously known as 'endothelial-derived relaxing factor', is released from endothelial cells. It produces relaxation of vascular smooth muscle and vasodilatation, and is an inhibitor of platelet aggregation. Endotoxin causes a release of NO from the endothelium, and its solubility allows free diffusion.

2.117   CDE

Monopolar diathermy uses an alternating current at a frequency of 400 kHz to 10 MHz. Current passes down the diathermy forceps, which may be applied to surgical forceps holding tissue, causing a local heating effect (up to 1000 °C) through the patient to the patient plate electrode (which must be at least 70 cm^2 in size). Bipolar diathermy avoids the need for the patient plate, and it uses less power as the current passes down one limb of the forceps and back up the other. Bipolar diathermy may not be applied through surgical forceps and may not be used for cutting tissue down. Monopolar diathermy may be used in patients with a pacemaker, but should be used in short bursts of less than 2 seconds, and the diathermy circuit should be away from the site of the pacemaker. It is preferable to use bipolar diathermy in these patients. Diathermy burns are usually full thickness.

2.118   BCD

Anthropomorphic indices have been used to assess nutritional status, such as triceps skin-fold thickness and mid-arm muscle circumference. Other forms of assessment include: body mass index, biochemical tests (transferrin, retinal-binding protein, thyroid-binding prealbumin) and dynamometric methods (such as hand-grip strength testing). The serum albumin level alone is not a reliable indicator of nutritional state.

2.119   AD
Metabolic acidosis is characterised by a low arterial pH. The serum bicarbonate (HCO_3^-) concentration may or may not be reduced, depending on whether compensatory mechanisms are functioning. Causes of metabolic acidosis include hypovolaemia, diabetic ketoacidosis, ingestion of alcohol or salicylates, septicaemia, renal failure, tissue necrosis, loss of HCO_3^- and massive blood transfusions. HCO_3^- is the main extracellular buffer, whereas proteins and phosphates represent the main intracellular buffers. Compensation occurs by an increase in alveolar ventilation (respiratory) and an increase in hydrogen ion excretion and HCO_3^- reabsorption by the kidneys (renal). Treatment is aimed at correcting the underlying cause.

2.120   ABCD
Complications of TPN can be line-related or metabolic. Metabolic complications include: hyper/hypoglycaemia, -natraemia, -kalaemia and -calcaemia. Deficiencies in folate, zinc, phosphate, magnesium and vitamins may occur. Liver function tests may become deranged, and a fatty liver and gallbladder stasis may occur.

2.121   ADF
Vitamin B_{12} is almost exclusively absorbed in the terminal ileum. Although pernicious anaemia leads to vitamin B_{12} deficiency, this is a specific autoimmune condition characterised by gastric atrophy and autoantibodies to intrinsic factor (which is essential for vitamin B_{12} absorption). Iron is mainly absorbed in the duodenum and upper jejunum. Folate is absorbed in the jejunum, and therefore deficiency does not occur after ileal resection. Bile salts are normally reabsorbed in the terminal ileum as part of the enterohepatic circulation. In the absence of this recirculation, the bile-salt pool is decreased and the solubility of cholesterol in the bile diminished. This can in turn lead to the formation of gallstones. Increased faecal loss of bile salts will result in watery diarrhoea.

2.122   BCDE
The normal CVP range is 3–8 cmH_2O. A low or negative reading confirms a low circulating blood volume. The response of the CVP to a fluid challenge of colloid gives much information regarding the state of the circulation. A dehydrated patient's CVP will rise in response to a challenge but fall to the original value as the circulation vasodilates. A sustained rise indicates a well-filled patient, but an elevation of greater than 4 cmH_2O indicates overfilling or a failing myocardium.

A bolus of any intravenous fluid may produce a rise in the CVP reading but it will not necessarily be sustained. If the patient is dehydrated there will be a drop in the reading after the initial rise. A sustained CVP rise of > 4 cmH$_2$O may indicate that the patient is overfilled, but this value should clearly be looked at with the clinical picture in mind. There is a well-recognised incidence of allergic reaction to the gelatins, although this is rare.

2.123   A
On administration, 5% dextrose is isotonic but becomes hypotonic as the dextrose is metabolised. Although it is evenly distributed through all the fluid compartments, only a small amount stays within the intravascular space because it passes easily into the interstitial space. It contains 278 mmol/l dextrose and has a negligible calorific content (30 kcal (~125.7 J)/l). Type I respiratory failure may be caused by the infusion of 5% dextrose.

2.124   CDF
Metabolic acidosis is characterised by a low plasma pH and low bicarbonate ion concentration. It can be caused by the addition of acid or the removal of alkali from the body, or by failure of the kidneys to excrete acid. Vomiting causes a loss of acid and so will result in a metabolic alkalosis. Hyperaldosteronism (Conn's syndrome) will cause alkalosis, hypokalaemia and hypertension. Diabetic ketoacidosis and renal failure will both cause a metabolic acidosis, as will septic shock (lactic acidosis).

2.125   ABE
Respiratory acidosis occurs when the Paco_2 is raised and the pH lowered. It is caused by hypoventilation. The causes can be divided into: airway obstruction, intrinsic lung disease, neuromuscular problems, chest wall problems and central respiratory-drive depression. Pulmonary embolus classically causes a respiratory alkalosis due to hyperventilation. Respiratory depression and failure may occur in a patient with a massive pulmonary embolus, so causing a respiratory acidosis.

2.126   ACD
Hyperbaric oxygen refers to an oxygen tension significantly greater than 1 kPa. An anaesthetic breathing circuit can only achieve approximately 1 kPa, so a pressurised chamber is required for the administration of hyperbaric oxygen. Typically, treatment involves several sessions of an hour or more. Among other effects, hyperbaric oxygen therapy is thought to improve oxygen delivery to cells and to reduce smoke-induced pulmonary oedema. Uses include the treatment of gas gangrene, necrotising fasciitis and carbon monoxide poisoning (though there has been conflicting evidence as to its efficacy). Exposure to more than 2 kPa tension of oxygen may cause acute oxygen toxicity, which can manifest as convulsions.

2.127   BCE
Haemorrhage is defined as an acute loss of circulating blood. The normal adult blood volume is approximately 5% of body weight (a 70-kg man has a 5-litre circulating blood volume), and in children it is approximately 8–9% of their body weight. The blood volume of obese patients is estimated using their ideal body weight, as their true weight gives an overestimation of blood volume. Tachycardia is the earliest measurable sign of haemorrhage.

2.128   ACDE
The causes of a PEA arrest include hypovolaemia, hypoxia, hypothermia, hyper/hypokalaemia, tension pneumothorax, cardiac tamponade, drug toxicity, electrolyte abnormalities, thromboembolism and mechanical obstruction. The treatment is basic life support, adrenaline (epinephrine; 1 mg per 3 minutes) and treatment of the underlying cause. Electric shock usually causes a ventricular fibrillatory arrest or occasionally an asystolic arrest.

2.129   ABCE
Hyperventilation causes a respiratory alkalosis. Rebreathing into a bag causes expired CO_2 to be stored in this reservoir and reabsorbed. Due to the physiological shifts, a change in the negatively charged protein buffers leads to a fall in free unbound calcium, thereby causing tetany.

2.130   ABD

The right ventricle is the most anterior chamber of the heart and most likely to be injured in penetrating trauma to the chest. Being anterior, it is best visualised by standard transthoracic echo. It is supplied by the right coronary artery and receives blood from the bronchial veins (remember the dual circulation of the lungs).

2.131   BCD

The most pronounced metabolic response to trauma begins to fall off approximately 24 hours after the surgery. The catabolism that accompanies trauma increases urea production and excretion. ADH levels rise as part of the endocrine response to stress. Increased serum cortisol leads to sodium and water retention.

2.132   ABDE

Theatre temperature is usually maintained between 22 °C and 24 °C but may need to be higher for neonatal surgery. Humidification and covering exposed surfaces will minimise heat loss. Anaesthesia obtunds the normal mechanisms of heat production, so the patient is vulnerable to hypothermia from conductive, convective and evaporative heat loss. Hypothermia also delays recovery from anaesthesia and postoperative shivering increases oxygen demands.

SECTION 3: PATHOLOGY – ANSWERS

3.1   AB
Metastatic calcification is defined as 'calcification occurring in otherwise normal tissue', and mainly affects the vessels, kidneys, lungs and gastric mucosa. Renal calculi are more likely to occur in patients with hyperparathyroidism. Squamous-cell carcinoma of the lung can produce parathyroid hormone and can therefore cause hyperparathyroidism. Rheumatoid arthritis is not associated with metastatic calcification. Rheumatoid nodules are made up of collagen, fibroblasts and macrophages. Calcification does occur in atherosclerosis and old tuberculous lesions, but this is dystrophic calcification.

3.2   ABCD
Hyperglycaemia results in increased vascular osmolarity and all its consequences. Poorly controlled diabetics have an increased risk of infection with unusual organisms owing to impairment of leucocyte phagocytic activity. There is no reported increased risk of haemorrhage.

3.3   All true
An embolism is the movement of solid, gaseous or immiscible material in flowing blood. A thromboembolus is a common type of embolus. Virchow's triad suggests that changes in blood components, the vessel wall or blood flow can trigger thrombus formation.

3.4   BE
Mast cells are distributed throughout the body and can usually be found in relation to small blood vessels in the connective tissue. They are involved in type I hypersensitivity reactions and the early phases of the acute inflammatory reaction. B lymphocytes are responsible for antibody production. In contrast, T lymphocytes are involved in cell-mediated immunity and are responsible for the presentation of antigens to the immune system, thereby playing a vital role in the up- or downregulation of the immune response. Phagocytic cells include polymorphonuclear leucocytes (particularly neutrophils), monocytes and tissue macrophages. Kupffer cells are part of the reticuloendothelial system involved in phagocytosis.

3.5   ACD

Captopril (an ACE inhibitor) and spironolactone (an aldosterone antagonist) may cause hyperkalaemia. In Conn's syndrome, there is excessive production of aldosterone which causes sodium retention and potassium loss. In diabetes insipidus, there is haemodilution, owing to water retention caused by excessive ADH. Excessive loss of potassium-rich secretions by a villous adenoma can lead to hypokalaemia.

3.6   CDE

Any cause of acidosis due to lowered bicarbonate (severe renal failure, ketoacidosis, lactic acidosis) will cause an altered distribution of potassium (hyperkalaemia). Suxamethonium chloride is a depolarising muscle relaxant, mimicking acetylcholine at the neuromuscular junction. It produces a transient rise in plasma potassium and creatinine phosphokinase concentrations.

3.7   AC

Diathermy uses the heating effect of electrical current. Although diathermy can be used in a patient with a pacemaker, the pad of the monopolar diathermy should be positioned well away from the pacemaker. Bipolar diathermy does not interfere with pacemakers and may be more suitable.

3.8   C

Metabolic alkalosis is characterised by a primary rise in the extracellular HCO_3^- concentration with a consequent fall in hydrogen ion concentration. Causes include loss of unbuffered hydrogen ion as in gastric aspiration, vomiting with pyloric stenosis, mineralocorticoid excess (Cushing's syndrome, Conn's syndrome) and potassium depletion. It is not usually a feature of vomiting if the pylorus is patent, as there is additional loss of HCO_3^- secretion from the upper intestine. In salicylate overdose, there is a mixed acid–base disorder of respiratory alkalosis and metabolic acidosis. A pancreatic fistula would cause a metabolic acidosis due to the loss of HCO_3^-. Acute renal failure leads to metabolic acidosis and hyperventilation.

3.9   ABCD

Pneumatic calf compression is used intraoperatively to reduce the incidence of DVT. Its effect is above and beyond that of TED stockings and subcutaneous heparin. The oral contraceptive pill should be stopped 4 weeks before surgery. Prolonged surgical procedures, due to increased immobility, will increase the incidence of DVT. Malignant disease has a strong association with venous thrombosis and in some cases may precede presentation of the cancer.

3.10   A

If possible, hypertension needs to be corrected before elective surgery in all patients, as it increases the risk of myocardial complications and stroke. Hypertension is defined as 160/90 mmHg (WHO definition). However, the presence of hypertension should not delay an emergency operation as the risks of delay will outweigh the dangers of an elevated blood pressure. Nevertheless, intraoperative lowering and control of blood pressure can be performed with sodium nitroprusside or esmolol.

3.11   ACEF

The non-microbial factors influencing the incidence of postoperative infection include: dead/damaged tissue within a wound; an excessive use of diathermy; and mass ligature. Face masks contribute little to the prevention of wound infection. Excessive pressure or tension in the tissues may impair the circulation of both blood and lymph. Inadequate haemostasis results in 'dead space', haematoma or seroma formation, which provide a favourable nidus for bacterial growth. A patient with well-controlled diabetes mellitus is no more susceptible to infection than non-diabetic patients. Steroids and ciclosporin suppress the host's response to infection by depressing antibody function, diminishing phagocytic activity and inhibiting new capillary formation.

3.12   CE

Occupationally acquired HIV infection in health workers occurs as a result of sharps injury, with hollow needles carrying a much greater risk. The overall risk of transmission of HIV infection is about 0.36% of all needlestick injuries from HIV-positive patients. At 6–12 weeks following HIV infection, there is a rise in antigen titre but no detectable antibody. At 3 months, 85% of HIV-infected patients mount an antibody response and their antigen levels fall. In HIV infection the CD4 (receptors found on helper T cells and macrophages) count falls. Hepatitis B virus is nearly 30 times more infectious than HIV.

3.13   CDE

Haematogenous infection from a primary focus elsewhere in the body is the commonest cause of osteomyelitis in neonates and children. Although this mode of infection can occur in adults, the commonest cause in this age group is following a compound fracture. *Staphylococcus* is the commonest organism in all age groups. In children, streptococci and Gram-negative organisms are found less commonly. In adults, a variety of organisms may be found but staphylococci predominate.

The treatment of osteomyelitis consists of analgesia, antibiotics and rest. If this fails, the abscess is drained through drill holes and the limb rested in a splint or plaster cast for several weeks.

3.14   BCE

Tourniquets should not be applied for longer than 1.5 hours and the pressure should not exceed 300 mmHg. If the tourniquet needs to be used for longer, an interval of 5 minutes should be allowed before re-applying pressure. The most common effect on peripheral nerves is neuropraxia. Mechanical effects of compression and ischaemia cause focal demyelination. 'Axonotmesis' means disruption of the axons while the nerve sheath remains intact.

3.15   CDE

The Nd-YAG (neodymium-yttrium aluminium garnet) laser penetrates tissue deeply (3–5 mm). It is useful for coagulating large tissue volumes, being especially useful in the ablation of exophytic oesophageal carcinoma, in controlling intestinal haemorrhage and in the treatment of low-grade bladder cancer. Safety measures are of paramount importance. There should be a designated area for laser use with a nominated user list. Adequate eye protection is required for users and patients at all times during laser procedures.

3.16   AE

Keloid scars extend beyond the previous wound (hypertrophic scars are confined to the wound). Keloid is most common on the sternum and deltoid area. Re-excision usually leads to a recurrence unless steroids (triamcinolone) are injected locally to reduce the scar formation. Pressure dressings work well, but the use of subcuticular sutures will not reduce keloid formation.

3.17   CFG

Mycobacterium tuberculosis hominis is the commonest causal organism for pulmonary tuberculosis in humans, and this is usually spread by air droplets. *Mycobacterium tuberculosis bovis* predominantly causes gastrointestinal tuberculosis, and is usually spread by the ingestion of infected milk. The hypersensitivity reaction is mediated by T lymphocytes, which liberate lymphokines. The Gohn focus refers to the initial site of infection in a non-immune individual. It is usually located in the subpleural, well-aerated regions of the lung (the upper lobe and upper part of the lower lobe).

3.18   D

Actinomycetes are Gram-positive microaerophilic bacteria, present as part of the normal flora of the mouth, lower gut and female genital tract. It is therefore an endogenous infection. The commonest site of actinomycosis infection is cervicofacial (about 50% of cases). Other sites of infection include the abdomen, thorax and female genital tract. The commonest organism producing infection is *Actinomyces israelii*, though *Actinomyces propionica* is occasionally responsible. Culture of the organism is slow, and it takes a week or more to produce positive cultures. The discharge contains characteristic sulphur granules.

3.19   ABC

HIV is a retrovirus, and definitive diagnosis is made by Western blotting. More recently, polymerase chain reaction (PCR) techniques have been used. HIV is present in high titre in the blood of asymptomatic carriers, and in many asymptomatic HIV-positive patients. The risk of seroconversion in someone following a needlestick injury from an HIV-positive patient is about 0.03%, and from a hepatitis B-positive patient it is approximately 30%. Hepatitis B is therefore potentially more infectious following a needlestick injury than HIV. The risk of infection from an HIV-positive individual is also dependent on the viral load of that individual.

3.20   BD

Hydatid disease is caused by the tapeworm *Echinococcus granulosus.* The intermediate host is the sheep. Dogs become infested by eating sheep offal and subsequently pass tapeworm eggs in their stool, which in turn contaminate their fur. This leads to accidental human ingestion. Therefore, humans act as an accidental intermediate host. Emergent embryos pass through the intestinal wall into the portal system and liver, and to other organs, where they develop into hydatid cysts. Hepatic lesions are often asymptomatic and discovered by chance on investigation of other problems. Diagnosis should be made on serological testing or from the typical appearances of cyst septation and daughter cysts on computed tomography. Needle biopsy is associated with the risk of anaphylaxis and dissemination of infection.

3.21   All true

The constituents of surgical equipment vary and hence different instruments will require different sterilisation techniques. Plastics and rubber can tolerate moisture, but may melt or become deformed by the extremes of heat, as with steam sterilisation or autoclaving. Gas sterilisation is used for delicate instruments that may otherwise corrode using the chemical technique. Dry-heat sterilisation is appropriate for equipment that can tolerate heat, but not moisture, or those that are not well penetrated by steam. Steam autoclaving is quick and effective, particularly for metal instruments and is commonly used to re-sterilise contaminated instruments if required quickly during a surgical procedure.

3.22   CE

Clostridium difficile infection is usually detected by identification of the cytotoxin. Gram staining of faeces is unhelpful in detecting the organism as it cannot distinguish *C. difficile* from many of the other gut organisms. The first step in treatment is cessation of the precipitating antibiotic(s). The two principal therapies are oral vancomycin 125 mg tds for 7–10 days or oral metronidazole 400 mg tds for 7–10 days. There is some evidence that oral vancomycin may be clinically more effective than metronidazole. Complications of *C. difficile* infection include electrolyte disturbances, paralytic ileus and, if pancolitis develops, toxic megacolon, perforation and endotoxic shock.

3.23   AE

Clostridium difficile infections have increased sixfold in the past few years. The ability of *C. difficile* to induce disease depends on the fact that the bacterium must be ingested into the colonic flora, and then become established. This usually occurs because the normal flora is disturbed. Disturbance of colonic flora is usually due to antibiotics, but chemotherapy (anti-neoplastic) drugs can also cause *C. difficile* infections. Third-generation cephalosporins (such as ceftazidime) are strongly associated with *C. difficile* infection. Diarrhoea usually starts within a few days, but up to 1–2 months may elapse before symptoms occur.

3.24   ABD

Actinomycosis is very sensitive to penicillin (the antibiotic of choice). However, infection is frequently found in association with other bacteria, and therefore it is advisable to treat the patient with metronidazole as well. Pus requires appropriate drainage or excisional surgery together with antibiotics.

3.25   AD

There is good evidence that chronic hepatitis B and C infections increase the risk of developing hepatocellular carcinoma. The acute illness of hepatitis C virus infection is generally less severe than that of hepatitis A or B viruses. Patients rarely become jaundiced and there is a less marked rise in enzymes.

3.26   AE

The risk of postsplenectomy sepsis is reduced by pneumococcal and HiB (*Haemophilus influenzae* type B) vaccination, as well as by maintenance prophylactic oral antibiotics (penicillin or amoxicillin). The vaccinations should be administered at least 2 weeks before splenectomy. The meningococcal vaccine is presently recommended only for those patients travelling to endemic areas or for those who are immunocompromised.

3.27   BCDEG

Hydatid disease is caused by *Echinococcus granulosus*. This disease occurs when humans ingest the embryos of the dog tapeworm. Human infection with *E. granulosus* frequently occurs in early childhood by direct contact with infected dogs or by eating uncooked or improperly washed vegetables contaminated with canine faeces. Embryo dissemination occurs to the liver (60%), lungs (20%), kidneys (3%) and brain (1%). Complications include epilepsy (from the space-occupying effect of the cysts) and peritonitis due to rupture of the cyst.

3.28   ABE

Interferon and interleukin-2 enhance the cytotoxic activity of natural killer cells, which play a major role in the destruction of malignant cells, virally infected cells and some normal cells, without prior sensitisation.

3.29   BCE

Immunocompromise will delay wound healing and increase the risk of postoperative complications such as wound infection and breakdown. AIDS patients have a high incidence of anorectal sepsis but undergo the same treatment for anorectal sepsis as non-AIDS patients. Pyomyositis presents with pain, tenderness and swelling, with overlying skin being smooth and shiny, thereby mimicking an abscess.

3.30   A

At present, there is no available vaccine against HIV. Patients do not need to be barrier-nursed. Hepatitis B is nearly 30 times more infectious than HIV. The risk of transmission of HIV is related to the depth of injury and the amount of blood and viral concentration load. Hollow needles potentially contain more blood, and hence virus, so the risk of transmission is higher. HIV survives for approximately 72 hours on fomites.

3.31   A

The internal organs of the body are free of commensal bacteria, apart from the alimentary tract, upper respiratory tract and oropharynx, genital tract, skin, external auditory meatus and conjunctiva.

3.32   BCDE

Staphylococcus aureus produces haemolysins, fibrinolysin, hyaluronidase (may assist spread of infection), leucocidin (destroys polymorphonuclear leucocytes), coagulase, enterotoxin (heat-stable proteins causing vomiting), toxic-shock syndrome toxin (related to enterotoxins) and epidermolytic toxins (cause splitting of epidermis and blister formation).

3.33   ACE

Acute inflammation is characterised by the presence of neutrophils. Neutrophils initially marginate, adhere to endothelial cells and then actively migrate between these cells. Neutrophils migrate in response to chemical mediators such as histamine, lysosomal compounds, prostaglandins, leukotrienes (especially leukotriene B4), 5-HT and lymphokines. C5a, C6 and C7 of the complement cascade are chemo-attractant to neutrophils. In acute inflammation neutrophils survive for only 24–48 hours, after which they are replaced by monocytes. Bradykinin is a chemical mediator of pain and a vasodilator. Chronic inflammation is characterised by the presence of macrophages, giant cells, fibroblasts, epithelioid cells and lymphocytes, but few or no neutrophils. Colony-stimulating factors can stimulate the production of leucocytes and megakaryocytes and may have a role in haemopoiesis.

3.34   A

Colloids such as Gelofusine® may cause anaphylaxis on rare occasions. Intestinal fluid contains large amounts of potassium and sodium and so colloids would be an inadequate fluid replacement. Crystalloids would therefore be more suitable. Whole blood is very rarely used except, perhaps, in trauma situations. Gelofusine® contains potassium and calcium, and for this reason should not be mixed with blood in a giving set as clotting will occur. Normal saline contains 154 mmol/l of sodium and 154 mmol/l of chloride.

3.35   BCD

Asplenic patients are at an increased risk of overwhelming sepsis caused by capsulated organisms such as *Streptococcus pneumoniae, Neisseria meningitidis* and *Haemophilus influenzae*. At present in the UK, vaccination is recommended against *Haemophilus* and *Pneumococcus* spp. This reduces the risk of infection and ideally should be given 2 weeks before surgery. Prophylactic oral antibiotics are effective in preventing postsplenectomy sepsis, which carries a 50% mortality. The antibiotic of choice is penicillin, but erythromycin is indicated in cases of allergy.

3.36   BCDE

Feeding by the enteral route is nutritionally, immunologically and metabolically superior to feeding using the parenteral route. Enteral nutrition provides a degree of protection against stress ulceration. The presence of nutrients in the upper small bowel stimulates the release of gut peptide hormones – it is by this mechanism that enteral nutrition promotes biliary flow and prevents cholestasis. A low nasogastric aspirate (< 250–300 ml/24 h) is the most appropriate prompt to initiate feeding.

3.37   ABD

Postoperative hypoxaemia in its episodic form can occur up to 3 days postoperatively. Although it is more common following narcotic infusions than with bolus doses, it does not occur with regional anaesthesia. Upper abdominal incisions are painful and patients often fail to make full respiratory incursions if analgesia is inadequate.

3.38   ABD

Steroids are associated with osteoporosis and also with avascular necrosis of bone – of the femoral head for example. Mineralocorticoid side effects include hypertension, hypernatraemia, hypokalaemia and water retention. Glucocorticoid side effects include diabetes, mental disturbances (usually depression or a serious paranoid state), Cushing's syndrome and obesity. Topical steroid use on eyes may lead to cataract formation. Hepatotoxicity and bone marrow suppression are seen with azathioprine use.

3.39   BDEFG

Excess steroids lead to hypernatraemia and hypokalaemia due to their mineralocorticoid effects on the distal convoluted tubule, namely sodium and water retention and potassium loss. Pyrexia leads to water loss and hence hypernatraemia. Irrigation during TURP may lead to excessive water absorption (the TURP syndrome). Small bowel obstruction, diarrhoea and vomiting can all cause hyponatraemia.

3.40   AB

Absorption of irrigating fluids can lead to the so-called 'TURP syndrome', causing metabolic acidosis, hyponatraemia, hypertension (from water overload) and confusion (from cerebral oedema), as well as a clotting abnormality due to the release of thromboplastins from the prostate. Hyperglycaemia may occur if dextrose irrigation is used. Glycine in the irrigation fluid can cause temporary blindness. Other symptoms include vomiting, headache, fatigue, weakness, muscle twitching and coma.

3.41   BC

The laboratory findings in haemolytic anaemia include the biochemical markers of increased red cell breakdown: unconjugated hyperbilirubinaemia; increased excretion of urobilinogen in the urine; and stercobilinogen in the faeces. Haptoglobins normally eliminate free haemoglobin in the plasma – in the presence of haemolysis they characteristically become saturated and are absorbed by reticuloendothelial cells. Hyperbilirubinaemia may lead to pigment gallstones. Increased red cell turnover leads to marrow hyperplasia and increased production of reticulocytes, leading to an increased mean cell volume.

3.42   AE

Excessive crystalloid administration results in: increased filtration pressure; reduced colloid osmotic pressure; and increased capillary permeability. The end result is interstitial and intra-alveolar oedema, promoting the development of ARDS. Initial volume expansion is more quickly achieved with colloid than with crystalloid. Neither colloid nor crystalloid administration prevents a fall in the haematocrit level following blood loss. Stored blood has a low pH and infusion may exacerbate an existing acidosis. Stored blood is also high in potassium and low in clotting factors and functioning platelets. Blood is the fluid of choice to replace continuing haemorrhage and hypotension. Bleeding sites need to be urgently identified and controlled.

3.43   ABC

Third-space loss is the temporary internal loss of extracellular fluid into a space that does not participate in the normal transport of nutrients or waste products. In moderately major operations, such as cholecystectomy, such a loss would be approximately 3 ml/kg/hour. In more extensive operations, such as aortic aneurysm repair, third-space fluid loss could initially be 10–20 ml/kg/hour. Dextrose-saline is a hypotonic solution, so when the dextrose is metabolised it increases the free-water content and so leads to hyponatraemia. Balanced salt solutions should be used to replace third-space losses. Transcellular losses that might be measured include ascites, pleural effusions and intraintestinal losses.

3.44   ABC

Cytotoxic T cells recognise foreign transplant antigens and have a major role in graft rejection. IgE is involved in the allergic response of atopic dermatitis. IgA is involved in the protection of mucosal surfaces.

3.45   ABD

Microcytic anaemia is characteristic of iron deficiency and is usually associated with chronic bleeding from the gut or with menorrhagia. Microcytic anaemia may occur in α- or β-thalassaemia and in sideroblastic anaemia (defect in haem synthesis). Hereditary haemochromatosis is a disorder of iron absorption characterised by iron overload and has no direct haematological manifestations. The anaemia of chronic renal failure is normocytic.

3.46   BCD

FFP contains all the non-cellular components of blood, including all clotting factors, immunoglobulin, albumin and other plasma proteins. Although FFP contains some fibrinogen, in certain situations (such as severe hypofibrinogenaemia associated with disseminated intravascular coagulation), it is usual to supplement FFP with cryoprecipitate which has a higher fibrinogen concentration. FFP is supplied as 150–200-ml units separated from a single whole-blood donation; or, in some centres, as a 300-ml unit obtained from a single-donor plasmapheresis. Units are stored at −30 °C for up to 1 year. FFP should be thawed in a waterbath in the transfusion laboratory and administered within 4 hours, usually at a dose of 12–15 ml/kg. Repeated transfusion should be prescribed according to the results of a post-transfusion coagulation screen. Donor FFP may contain anti-A or anti-B antibodies, which can sometimes cause dramatic haemolysis of recipient red cells. FFP is therefore usually issued as ABO-compatible.

3.47   DE

Haemophilia A is a sex-linked inherited disorder characterised by a complete or partial deficiency of factor VIII. Heterozygous female carriers have a factor VIII level of approximately 50%, although some individuals have sufficiently low levels to cause clinical symptoms. Severe disease (factor VIII < 1%) is characterised by painful joint and muscle bleeds that eventually lead to a chronic arthropathy. Rarer manifestations include pseudotumour formation following muscle bleeds, nerve entrapment, compartment syndromes, haematuria and post-traumatic intracranial bleeds. Significant mortality arises from replacement therapy associated with HIV, hepatitis B and hepatitis C infection. Haemophilia B is a sex-linked disorder arising from deficiency of factor IX. The clinical pattern is similar to haemophilia A.

Section 3: Pathology – Answers

3.48 ABCF

The daily folic acid requirement is 50 mg, but increased amounts are needed during pregnancy. The storage capacity for folic acid is sufficient for about 80–100 days and it is mainly stored in the liver. Any malnutritional state such as anorexia or alcoholism will predispose to folic acid deficiency. Other causes include coeliac disease, tropical sprue, Crohn's disease and drugs such as phenytoin, trimethoprim and methotrexate.

3.49 ABD

Postoperative DVT is confirmed in 30% of patients when no prophylactic anticoagulant measures are taken. Factor V Leiden is a mutation that causes resistance to activated protein C and is found in 60% of idiopathic DVTs. Other inherited causes of an increased risk of DVT include antithrombin III deficiency and protein S and C deficiencies.

3.50 BDE

Laboratory features of iron deficiency anaemia include: decreased serum iron concentration; a raised TIBC; and absent iron in both the marrow and erythroblasts. Tissue oxygen delivery is dependent on haemoglobin and therefore will be affected. Anaemia does not cause a shift in the oxygen dissociation curve. The presence of a posterior cricoid web and iron deficiency is a recognised association (Plummer–Vinson syndrome). Treatment with aspirin can cause gastritis, and associated haemoglobin loss over a prolonged period can deplete iron stores.

3.51 BDE

Fibrin dissolution can be reduced by tranexamic acid, which acts by inhibiting plasminogen activation and fibrinolysis. It is useful in cases where it is difficult to stop haemorrhage directly, as in prostatectomy. Epsilon-aminocaproic acid also inhibits the fibrinolytic system. Protein C is an important natural inhibitor of blood clotting. Factor XII acts upon prekallikrein to form kallikrein, which activates the fibrinolytic system through the intrinsic pathway. Tissue plasminogen activator (tPA) is produced by endothelial cells. It binds to fibrin, converting fibrin-bound plasminogen to plasmin, which in turn degrades to fibrin.

3.52   AC
Vitamin B_{12} is involved in the red cell maturation process and haemopoiesis, but not in haemoglobin synthesis directly. In deficient states, megaloblastic erythropoiesis results. Vitamin B_{12} cannot be absorbed except in the presence of intrinsic factor, a glycoprotein secreted by the stomach. The intrinsic factor-vitamin B_{12} complex is selectively absorbed in the terminal ileum. Stores of vitamin B_{12} are very great in the liver. A vitamin B_{12} deficiency takes approximately 5 years to develop.

3.53   A
Aspirin and clopidogrel are both antiplatelet agents and have no effect on blood cross-matching. Warfarin increases the international normalised ratio (INR) by inhibiting the production of vitamin K-dependent factors II, VII, IX and X, but it does not affect cross-matching and compatibility testing *per se*. Gelofusine® too does not affect blood cross-matching, which is one of the advantages of using this fluid in resuscitation.

3.54   CE
Human albumin solution is available in 20-g units, either as 400 ml of a 5% solution or 100 ml of a 20% solution. The 20% solution is hyperoncotic and will therefore expand the plasma volume by more than the volume infused. The 5% solution has a sodium content of 130–150 mmol/litre and may precipitate hypernatraemia. Human albumin is manufactured from large pools of donations and is subjected to virus-inactivation procedures, hence the viral safety is excellent. The freeze-dried product has a long shelf-life at room temperature. Clinical indications include the treatment of hypoproteinaemic oedema with nephrotic syndrome and ascites in liver failure. There is no evidence that a 5% human albumin solution is superior to colloids in acute volume replacement.

3.55   BE

Autologous transfusion of preoperatively donated blood is a useful technique that minimises the hazards of infection transmission and alloantibody stimulation. It is particularly useful in patients who already have multiple alloantibodies and who are difficult to cross-match. The procedure still carries a small risk of a transfusion reaction, either through bacterial contamination of the donor units or by human error in transfusing the wrong blood. Patients who are unable to tolerate large venesections (such as children and those with pre-existing anaemia, cardiac or respiratory disease) or those with HIV or hepatitis B or C are unsuitable. Donations must be made at not less than weekly intervals and not within 4 days of surgery. The finite shelf-life of stored blood therefore limits the maximum collection to 4–5 units.

3.56   AF

Coagulation is initiated *in vivo* by the exposure of circulating factor VII to tissue factor, which in turn activates factor X (extrinsic pathway). Activated factor X subsequently sustains and amplifies the pathway by activating more factor VII and by activating factors XII, XI, IX, VIII and V (intrinsic pathway). Both pathways generate more activated factor X, which, in sufficient concentration, converts prothrombin to thrombin – this in turn converts fibrinogen to fibrin (common pathway), so producing a fibrin clot. The process is completed by factor XIII which stabilises the fibrin clot.

Clotting factors are predominantly synthesised in the liver – factor II, VII, IX and X synthesis being vitamin K-dependent. The coagulation cascade is inhibited *in vivo* by antithrombin III and the protein S and C pathways. Deficiency of these proteins therefore predisposes to thrombosis. Deficiency of the extrinsic, intrinsic and common pathway factors predisposes to haemorrhage, with the exception of factor XII deficiency, which is asymptomatic.

3.57   ACDE

DIC is characterised by the simultaneous activation of the coagulation and fibrinolytic pathways, which results in the consumption and depletion of platelets and clotting factors. Clinical presentation is usually with haemorrhage, but thrombosis may occur and tissue ischaemia may be apparent if the coagulation pathways are dominant. Common causes of DIC include sepsis, malignancy (especially adenocarcinoma), trauma and obstetric emergencies. Laboratory features include prolongation of all clotting times and a progressively falling platelet count and fibrinogen concentration. Increasing fibrin degradation products (FDP) indicate activation of the fibrinolytic system, and, in the context of the other laboratory abnormalities, support a diagnosis of DIC. An isolated raised FDP level is seen in other conditions, including liver disease, and may cause diagnostic confusion. Treatment involves intensive blood-product support with correction of the underlying cause.

3.58   CE

The intravenous giving set should be removed but the cannula retained as intravenous access is required. The patient should be given large quantities of intravenous fluids to promote a urine output of > 1.5 ml/kg/hour. Furosemide (frusemide) should be given to promote diuresis, and a central line should be inserted if the patient remains oliguric. 100 ml of 20% mannitol are recommended for 'renal protection'. Hyperkalaemia and DIC may both occur and require specific treatment.

3.59   BCDE

A raised mean cell volume occurs with macrocytosis associated with the dietary deficiency or malabsorption of vitamin B_{12} and folate, liver disease (especially associated with alcohol abuse), hypothyroidism, myelodysplasia and after exposure to some drugs (cytotoxics). Vitamin B_{12} is found exclusively in animal products and deficiency is a hazard of veganism. Conditions such as haemolytic anaemia or recovery from acute haemorrhage lead to an increased erythropoietic drive and hence the appearance of reticulocytes in the circulation. This may manifest as a raised mean cell volume because reticulocytes have a higher cell volume than mature red cells. Iron deficiency is associated with microcytosis.

3.60   BDE
APTT measures the integrity of the intrinsic and common coagulation pathways. Hence, it is sensitive to a deficiency of factors VIII, IX, XI, XII and to a lesser extent factors V, X and prothrombin. The APTT is prolonged in patients on warfarin, except in the very early stages, owing to impaired synthesis of the vitamin K-dependent factors II, VII, IX and X. Intravenous heparin potentiates the activity of the endogenous anticoagulant antithrombin III and prolongs the APTT by inhibiting the intrinsic and common pathway factors. Low-molecular-weight heparin selectively inhibits factor Xa and at therapeutic doses has little or no effect on the APTT. Thromboprophylaxis with subcutaneous heparin does not usually prolong the APTT. Lupus anticoagulant is an example of a coagulation factor inhibitor that has affinity to factors in the intrinsic pathway. The presence of a lupus anticoagulant impairs the function of these factors and so prolongs the APTT.

3.61   AB
Petechial haemorrhages are usually associated with vascular or platelet disorders. Coagulation disorders are typically associated with haemarthrosis and muscle haematomas. Scurvy is usually associated with swollen spongy gums with spontaneous bruising, haemorrhage and perifollicular haemorrhages. However, vitamin C deficiency may cause petechial haemorrhages.

3.62   BDE
Thrombocytopenia is a common haematological abnormality, and usually arises from increased peripheral destruction of platelets in disorders such as immune thrombocytopenia, disseminated intravascular coagulation, hypersplenism or following heparin therapy. Thrombocytopenia may also occur in infiltrative bone marrow disorders such as carcinomatosis. Artefactual thrombocytopenia may result from platelet clumping *in vitro* following difficult venesection. Spontaneous bleeding in an afebrile patient with otherwise normal haemostasis is unlikely at platelet counts above 10×10^9/l. Thrombocytosis may indicate an acute phase response in sepsis, inflammatory disorders or malignancy. It is common for the platelet count to rise transiently after splenectomy.

3.63   BCDE

Coagulation is initiated *in vivo* by the interaction between tissue factor (TF) in the tissues and factor VII in the plasma. Anatomical separation of TF from the plasma prevents activation of the pathway, unless vascular integrity is breached. Alternatively, coagulation can be initiated if TF is pathologically expressed on vascular cells, as in malignancy, disseminated intravascular coagulation and inflammation. If TF and factor VII interact, the resultant complex activates factor X and so completes the extrinsic pathway. In turn, factor X activates small quantities of thrombin, that back-activates factors V, VIII, IX and X (intrinsic and common pathways) in the presence of anionic phospholipids on the surface of activated platelets. This provides amplification of the pathway by generating larger quantities of thrombin. Eventually, sufficient thrombin is formed to cleave fibrinogen to fibrin to form a thrombus. Coagulation is limited *in vivo* by the activation of the anticoagulants antithrombin III, protein S and protein C by thrombin.

3.64   BDE

Although acute haemolytic transfusions are almost exclusively caused by ABO incompatibility, haemolysis may also occur due to anti-Rh D, Rh E, Rh C and anti-Kell antibodies. In these cases, haemolysis occurs within the liver and spleen. The usual presentation is with fever, nausea and shivering, usually about an hour after transfusion. Alternatively, in parous women or previous recipients of transfusions, there may be undetectable pretransfusion antibodies that increase dramatically after re-exposure as a secondary antibody response. This may manifest as a delayed haemolytic transfusion reaction presenting 5–10 days after transfusion, with fever, a falling haemoglobin level, jaundice and haemoglobinuria. Fever and rigors occur in about 1–2% of red cell and platelet transfusions and may indicate a non-haemolytic febrile transfusion reaction. This is most common in parous women and those previously transfused. It represents a recipient antibody response to donor white cell antigens. Allergic reactions, ranging from mild urticaria to anaphylaxis, are usually due to an antibody response to donor plasma proteins.

3.65   All true

Graft-versus-host disease (GVHD) is a near-universally fatal condition caused by T lymphocytes in donor blood, and is characterised by fever, skin rash and gastrointestinal and liver dysfunction, starting 4–30 days after transfusion. GVHD is prevented by using gamma-irradiated blood products. Lymphocyte contaminants in red cell products have immunosuppressant activity even in immunocompetent recipients. There is some evidence that recurrence of malignancy and sepsis are more common in heavily transfused patients undergoing surgery for malignant disease. Iron overload is inevitable in patients on long-term transfusion programmes. This may manifest as hepatic cirrhosis, endocrine insufficiency or cardiomyopathy. Post-transfusion purpura is a potentially fatal disorder, which is due to the production of antibodies against foreign platelet antibodies after transfusion. Thrombocytopenia in the recipient occurs when these antibodies cross-react with the recipient's own platelets. In the United Kingdom, blood products are not screened for the human T-cell leukaemia viruses (HTLV-I and -II) and a small number of patients acquire the lifelong risk of T-cell leukaemia from transfusions each year.

3.66   ABCD

Massive blood transfusion is defined as replacement of the whole blood volume within 24 hours. Since red cell donations contain few platelets and low concentrations of coagulation factors, dilutional thrombocytopenia and coagulopathy can occur. Other sequelae include hypocalcaemia, hyperkalaemia and metabolic alkalosis. Correction of these biochemical and haematological abnormalities should be on an 'as needed' basis. Hypothermia is a recognised hazard and a blood warmer should be used routinely. ARDS is a well-recognised complication.

3.67   B

Cardiopulmonary bypass is often associated with thrombocytopenia and platelet dysfunction. It is usually combined with induced hypothermia to reduce tissue metabolic demand. Plasma coagulation factor levels drop due to haemodilution. Heparin is routinely used to prevent extracorporeal clotting in the oxygenerator. Protamine sulphate is used at the end of a bypass to neutralise the remaining circulating heparin.

3.68   ADE

PT measures the integrity of the extrinsic and common pathways of coagulation and is therefore sensitive to a deficiency or inhibition of factors II, V, VII and X. It is particularly sensitive to the global impairment of coagulation factor synthesis seen in severe liver disease or to vitamin K deficiency (impaired synthesis of factors II, VII, IX and X). Coagulation factor deficiencies which affect only the intrinsic pathway, such as haemophilia A (factor VIII deficiency), will not prolong the PT. PT is usually expressed as an international normalised ratio (INR) when monitoring oral anticoagulant dose. This allows standardisation of reagents between different laboratories.

3.69   All true

Inherited deficiencies or defects in components of the coagulation cascade with anticoagulant activity predispose to spontaneous and perioperative venous thrombosis. These include: antithrombin III, protein S and protein C deficiencies; and the factor V Leiden mutation. Acquired risk rises with increasing age, malignancy, a previous history of thrombosis, immobilisation, obesity, the combined oral contraceptive pill, hormone replacement therapy and pregnancy. Thrombosis also occurs more frequently in patients with sickle cell disease, inflammatory bowel disease and myeloproliferative disorders.

3.70   A

Warfarin is an orally active anticoagulant that rapidly depletes hepatic vitamin K by impairing its recycling. It acts by preventing the synthesis of the vitamin K-dependent factors II, VII, IX and X and therefore requires at least 48 hours to become effective. Although warfarin treatment will prolong both the APTT and the prothrombin time (PT), the PT is a more reliable index of anticoagulant activity. It is usual practice to express the PT as an international normalised ratio (INR) when measuring anticoagulation. Complications of treatment include bleeding and, rarely, skin necrosis. Warfarin has numerous interactions with other drugs, commonly antibiotics (which either reduce or enhance its bioavailability).

3.71   BCE

LMWHs are prepared by enzymatic degradation of unfractionated heparin, so reducing their mean molecular weight from 15 to 4–7 kDa. LMWHs therefore have a longer half-life than unfractionated heparin and better bioavailability after subcutaneous injection. Only a once-daily administration is required. LMWHs act predominantly by inhibiting factor Xa and, unlike unfractionated heparin, they have low antithrombin activity. Consequently, a patient may be adequately anticoagulated with an LMWH without prolongation of the APTT. Excretion is almost exclusively renal and so dose reduction is required in patients with renal failure.

3.72   BDE

von Willebrand's disease is the commonest inherited bleeding disorder in white populations and is usually autosomal dominant in inheritance. Affected individuals have reduced or dysfunctional von Willebrand factor (vWF), a protein normally present in platelets and endothelium. vWF stabilises factor VIII in the circulation and mediates platelet adhesion at the site of vascular injury. The associated laboratory abnormalities therefore include a prolonged APTT (due to reduced factor VIII), a normal prothrombin time and a prolonged bleeding time (platelet adhesion defect). Clinically, affected individuals usually show a mild bleeding tendency with epistaxis, easy bruising, menorrhagia and gingival bleeding. Although factor VIII levels are characteristically reduced, levels are rarely sufficiently low to cause haemarthroses, the hallmark of haemophilia A. Preoperative management usually involves treatment with desmopressin (which liberates platelet stores of vWF) or factor replacement with either intermediate-purity factor VIII or a specific vWF concentrate.

3.73   AB

Bleeding time is a global test of small-vessel haemostasis. It may be altered in thrombocytopenia, disorders of platelet function and collagen disorders affecting the vessel wall. However, the correlation with surgical bleeding is poor. Aspirin irreversibly inactivates platelets by inhibiting cyclo-oxygenase and therefore prolongs the bleeding time. Fibrinogen is manufactured in the liver and its synthesis is increased as part of the acute phase response. A reduced fibrinogen concentration may indicate a consumptive coagulopathy. The TT is a measure of the conversion of fibrinogen to fibrin and is therefore prolonged in hypofibrinogenaemia. Inhibitors of fibrin polymerisation – such as heparin, fibrin degradation products and severe hypoalbuminaemia – also prolong the TT. Heparin may cause significant prolongation of the TT at concentrations well below those needed to prolong the activated partial thromboplastin time.

3.74   BD

Following splenectomy there is an early thrombocytosis, usually peaking between 7 and 10 days. There are increased circulating Howell–Jolly bodies (DNA fragments of nuclear origin, normally present in < 2% of circulating red blood cells (RBCs)) and an increased proportion of target cells, sideroblasts (RBCs containing granules of free iron) and RBCs containing Heinz bodies (degraded haemoglobin, usually found in ageing RBCs). An early leucocytosis (usually neutrophils) is seen within hours and may last for several weeks. There is also increased platelet adhesiveness and platelet dysfunction.

3.75   BDE

Acute haemolytic transfusion reactions are the result of administration of ABO-incompatible blood: group A, B or AB to a group O recipient; group A or AB to a group B recipient; or group B or AB to a group A recipient. Human error outside the transfusion laboratory is the commonest cause. Clinically, the reaction can be recognised by the very rapid onset of agitation, flushing, pain at the venepuncture site, abdomen, flank or chest, a fever, hypotension, haemoglobinuria or haemoglobinaemia. This may be clinically indistinguishable from the effects of transfusing blood contaminated with Gram-negative organisms. Management should be the immediate cessation of transfusion, supportive measures and confirmation of the diagnosis with serological and haematological investigations.

3.76   ABDEG
Circulating fat globules > 10 mm in diameter and histological traces of fat emboli in the lungs occur in most adults after closed fractures of long bones. These fat emboli can impact not only in the lung microvasculature, but also in the brain. Fortunately, only a small number of patients develop the fat embolism syndrome. The source is thought to be the bone marrow. Early warning signs are a slight rise in temperature and pulse rate. Petechiae should be sought on the front and back of the chest, axilla and conjunctival folds. Fat droplets may be found not only in sputum, but also in urine, blood and CSF. Restlessness, drowsiness and even chest pain may occur. Some studies suggest that steroids can both prevent and treat the fat embolism syndrome.

3.77   ACDE
During the catabolic phase of the metabolic response to trauma, increased levels of ADH lead to water retention. Increased aldosterone levels lead to sodium retention. There is negative potassium balance in the first few days, although this rarely amounts to more than the average daily intake. Therefore, during the first couple of days post-trauma, water and salt requirements are likely to be less than normal and potassium supplements are not required. Gluconeogenesis in the liver is stimulated by cortisol, amino acids from the catabolism of muscle acting as the substrate, leading to a negative nitrogen balance, which may persist for up to 2 weeks in patients with severe burns. Among the haematological responses are thrombocytosis and neutrophilia.

3.78   BCE
Catecholamines are secreted by the adrenal medulla, and a decrease in atrial pressure stimulates ADH secretion by the Henry–Gauer reflex. Decreased PaO_2 stimulates chemoreceptors, and with increased ventilation (tidal ventilation) and reduced cardiac output there is an increase in $\dot{V}/\dot{Q}$ mismatch. The oxygen–haemoglobin dissociation curve shifts to the left.

3.79   All true
Fracture of the frontal skull can cause anosmia due to damage to the cribriform plate (olfactory nerve) and visual defects by damage to the orbit and optic chiasma. Discharge from the nose or ear may indicate leakage of CSF. Other indications of a basal skull fracture are: bruising over the mastoid bone (retroauricular ecchymoses, Battle's sign); periorbital ecchymosis ('racoon eyes'); and VIIth cranial nerve palsy.

3.80   ABCD

Extradural haematoma is associated with fracture and is usually the result of damage to the anterior part of the middle meningeal artery. The dura has strong attachments to the cranium along the suture lines and as a result, these attachments can limit the extent of the haematoma. Subdural haematomas tend to follow a contre-coup injury, whereas extradural haematoma typically occurs with a direct local impact (coup).

3.81   A

Tracheal stenosis following tracheostomy may occur at three possible sites: the level of the stoma; the level of the cuff; and at the tube tip. The incidence is approximately 10%. The standard approach is a 2-cm transverse incision 2 cm above the sternal notch. The thyroid isthmus may need to be tied as it lies over the second and third tracheal rings. This has no effect on the thyroid status of the patient. In adults, the tracheostomy is placed between the second and fourth tracheal rings, and in children at the second and third tracheal rings. The cough reflex is lost in someone with a tracheostomy and the patient is therefore unable to clear secretions from the tracheobronchial tree, so frequent suction is necessary.

3.82   EF

Chronic subdural haematomas are most commonly found in the older age groups. Chronic alcohol ingestion is also an associated factor due to the frequent incidence of falls. Chronic subdural haematomas are collections of altered blood and are most frequently triggered by minor trauma. The symptoms include progressive headache, failing intellect, hemiparesis and a fluctuating conscious level. Acute subdural haematoma is more commonly associated with anosmia and rhinorrhoea as there is usually a concomitant skull fracture.

3.83   ABC

Systemic features of the crush syndrome include hyperkalaemia, hypocalcaemia, myoglobinaemia, anuric renal failure and coagulopathy. This occurs as a result of ischaemia and subsequent muscle necrosis. Myoglobin and other breakdown products are released following muscle necrosis, thereby causing acute tubular necrosis. Haemoconcentration, oliguria and uraemia are well documented.

3.84 ACE

Tachycardia in response to haemorrhage may be absent in: the elderly; patients on β-blockers and calcium antagonists; patients with hypothermia; and patients who have a pacemaker. Infants will develop a tachycardia and the rate will be much higher than in adults. Athletes have a higher cardiac output and stroke volume but a lower resting pulse than the average population. The usual responses to hypovolaemia may not be manifest in athletes until a significant blood loss has occurred. Oxygen has no effect on this response.

3.85 CE

In the immediate aftermath of a traumatic insult to the body, a complex series of responses are set in motion. Underperfusion of the tissues leads to a decrease in metabolic rate and body temperature, and an increase in anaerobic metabolism with the formation of lactic acid and a secondary metabolic acidosis. Increased levels of catecholamines stimulate lipolysis and glycogenolysis, which lead to hyperglycaemia in the presence of decreased insulin levels; this hyperglycaemia is exacerbated by the conversion of lactic acid in the liver to glucose.

3.86 ACDE

Antidiuretic hormone (ADH), catecholamines and corticosteroids are elevated following trauma. This has the effect of conserving sodium and water and producing a hyperglycaemia.

3.87 ADG

The classical symptom triad of cardiac tamponade (Beck's triad) includes muffled heart sounds, distended neck veins and hypotension, and is seen in the majority of patients. Pulsus paradoxus is defined as a fall in systolic blood pressure of over 10 mmHg on inspiration. This only occurs in 1 in 10 cases of tamponade. In cardiac tamponade, the cardiac outline on CXR is classically globular. Charcot's triad refers to fever, jaundice and abdominal pain, and is suggestive of cholangitis. In severe haemorrhage, the CVP may not be elevated even in cardiac tamponade.

3.88 CD

Extradural haematomas are usually biconvex in appearance, whereas subdural ones are crescenteric. In contrast to subdural haematomas, extradural haematomas do not usually cross suture lines as the dura is normally very adherent to the cranium. Both subdural and extradural haematomas can cross the midline. Decreased attenuation of a haematoma is usually a feature of a chronic subdural haematoma (over 21 days old).

3.89   BD
Major burns are associated with splanchnic vasoconstriction on both the arteriolar and venular sides of the circulation. Curling's ulcers are stress ulcers related to major burns. They have a propensity to massive bleeding and have a poor prognosis.

3.90   ACD
Pulmonary ventilation–perfusion mismatch results from lung contusion, haematomas and alveolar collapse. Reduced ventilation results in hypercarbia. Hypovolaemia from blood loss and changes in intrathoracic pressure relationships (from tension or open pneumothoraces) clearly compromise oxygen exchange.

3.91   ACD
Major burns are associated with numerous complications, as are other forms of major trauma. Muscle loss/injury due to electrical burns may lead to myoglobinuria. Potassium levels tend to rise due to cellular damage and sodium levels can be raised or lowered owing to excessive or inadequate fluid resuscitation.

3.92   ACDE
Respiratory failure can be divided into type I and type II. Type I is where the PaO_2 is low and the Pco_2 is normal or low, and type II is where the PO_2 is low and the $Paco_2$ is high. In practical terms this occurs when the PO_2 is < 8 kPa and the $Paco_2$ > 7 kPa. Certainly, an inability to clear secretions would will lead to respiratory insufficiency. This often occurs after abdominal surgery (especially upper) when pain prevents deep inspiration and coughing, with subsequent basal atelectasis and retention of secretions. The symptoms of respiratory insufficiency include confusion, agitation and drowsiness. In pancreatitis, inflammatory mediators are released into the circulation and this can produce respiratory impairment through acute lung injury, which may progress to fulminant adult respiratory distress syndrome.

3.93   C
Following any trauma or sepsis there is a negative nitrogen balance. Metabolic rate increases and protein from muscle stores is mobilised for repair and energy, which results in increased urea production and a net nitrogen loss. This may be prolonged for many weeks if sepsis or multiorgan failure occurs.

3.94 ABCD
The pressure in the veins situated above the level of the right atrium is below that of the atmosphere, so when a wound involves the wall of such a vein, air may be sucked into it and pass into the circulation. It may also happen where positive pressure is used in venous or arterial catheterisation and in venous infusion of fluids. *C. perfringens* causes gas gangrene; hydrogen peroxide is used to irrigate wounds during debridement, and formation of gas emboli has been described.

3.95 AB
The risk factors for postoperative renal failure include sepsis, jaundice and hypotension. Jaundice is a well-known risk factor for developing renal failure, which may lead to the hepatorenal syndrome. Sepsis is one of the most common causes of acute renal failure in surgery. Benign prostatic hypertrophy leads to acute urinary retention, but does not lead to postoperative renal failure unless it is left untreated.

3.96 BCD
ARDS is the most extreme manifestation of acute lung injury. It produces diffuse alveolar shadows on CXR. Early radiographic signs are non-specific. The final common pathway of ARDS involves neutrophil activation, and the release of inflammatory mediators and free radicals causing increased alveolar permeability. ARDS should be managed in the ITU/HDU environment as rapid deterioration can occur requiring advanced circulatory support.

3.97 AC
Acute renal failure results in a metabolic acidosis. So, the blood pH and plasma bicarbonate level drop. To compensate, the respiratory rate increases and carbon dioxide levels are lowered. The biochemical features of ARF include a hyperkalaemia, hyponatraemia and elevated urea and creatinine. Phosphate is elevated and calcium lowered.

3.98   AB
Nitric oxide is a molecule with broad and diverse effects. It was first described in 1980 as a product of endothelial cells that causes vasorelaxation. This product was called endothelium-derived relaxing factor (EDRF) and was eventually shown to be nitric oxide. Nitric oxide is known to be produced by many cell types and to exert a wide range of biological effects. The physiological actions of nitric oxide include relaxation of gastrointestinal smooth muscle and bronchial smooth muscle, maintenance of vascular integrity, and inhibition of smooth muscle migration and proliferation. Endothelial nitric oxide also plays a critical role in haemostasis, making an important contribution to the normal inhibition of platelet function. Inhibition of platelet adhesion is a property of nitric oxide. Nitric oxide is also an important determinant of blood cell flow and is thought to be involved in immune and inflammatory responses via its production in macrophages, lymphocytes and neutrophils. Nitric oxide is synthesised by a family of enzymes, the nitric oxide synthetases.

3.99   BCD
Fluid resuscitation is essential to ensure that the patient is adequately filled, with a blood pressure sufficient for renal perfusion (prerenal failure). All nephrotoxic drugs should be stopped. The initial management is supportive; dialysis is used for chronic renal failure. In the emergency setting, haemofiltration is used when there is fluid overload, hyperkalaemia (> 6.0 mmol/l) or metabolic acidosis (pH < 7.2 and deteriorating base excess) resistant to treatment.

3.100   BCD
Dissection of the ascending aorta (DeBakey types I and III) may disrupt the ostia of the coronary arteries and so cause cardiac ischaemia and infarction. Distortion of the aortic valve may occur, leading to valvular incompetence. Rupture into the pericardium can cause tamponade, although this is rare.

3.101   ABCE
The causes of ARDS can broadly be divided into direct and indirect insults to the lung. Direct insults include lung contusion, aspiration and pneumonia. Indirect insults include massive blood transfusion, pancreatitis and fat embolus. Renal failure may be associated with ARDS, especially in the presence of multiorgan failure. It is, however, not a cause of ARDS.

3.102   B

Emergency tracheostomy is a formal operation and should be carried out under controlled circumstances under general anaesthetic. However, percutaneous tracheostomy is performed under local anaesthetic in some centres. It is useful in enabling adequate toilet of the lungs and the reduction in dead space may aid weaning from ventilation. Anatomical dead space of the respiratory tract refers to all the areas not involved in gas exchange, such as the oropharynx.

3.103   BCE

By adequately inflating the lungs, artificial ventilation will help to prevent the collapse of small airways. However, overforceful ventilation pressures may cause a pneumothorax and subsequent surgical emphysema. The use of positive end-expiratory pressure to reduce alveolar closing may lead to a positive intrathoracic pressure, which in turn may reduce venous return to the heart, so reducing cardiac output. Artificial ventilation can be used to induce hypocarbia and so reduce intracranial pressure. Acute gastric distension may occur with ventilation, and this usually responds well to the insertion of a nasogastric tube.

3.104   AB

Pain often causes an elevation of systemic arterial pressure via sympathetic nervous system stimulation. This is often related to the wound or, occasionally, to urinary retention. The volatile anaesthetic agents do not cause hypertension and epidurals most frequently cause postoperative hypotension due to sympathetic blockade and loss of vasomotor tone.

3.105   EF

Hyperkalaemia produces peaked T waves, slows conduction time and inhibits the myocardium, so leading to ventricular standstill. Acidosis causes a shift of potassium from the intracellular to the extracellular compartment. The pancreatic juices are rich in potassium and the presence of a high-output fistula may lead to hypokalaemia.

3.106   AE

In acute respiratory failure the PaO_2 falls and the $PaCO_2$ rises with a consequent drop in pH. In chronic respiratory failure, the serum bicarbonate concentration increases to correct the acidaemia. The rise of bicarbonate concentration in the CSF renders the respiratory centre in the brainstem insensitive to hypercarbia but not to hypoxia. So, a hypoxic respiratory drive is the predominant mechanism and is the only stimulus to increase the ventilation rate.

3.107   BCD

ARF occurs in about 30% of critically ill patients. Loss of renal function leads to a 60% increase in mortality and morbidity. The common causes of ARF include postoperative hypovolaemia, congestive cardiac failure, radiocontrast and drugs (aminoglycosides, NSAIDs). Only 20% of ARF is drug-induced. In 60% of cases, ARF is potentially avoidable, as it is the result of fluid or drug mismanagement. The histological appearance of the kidney bears little relevance to the level of renal dysfunction – a severe functional renal deficit can occur with minimal histological changes. The proximal tubule is the segment that is most susceptible to injury and reflects the relative hypoxia in the outer medulla and inner cortex.

3.108   ACEF

Changes in cellular metabolism associated with shock include accumulation of lactic acid and reduced ATP production due to anaerobic metabolism. Changes in membrane function result in the passage of sodium into cells and the passage of potassium out of cells. Lysosomal fragmentation occurs as a result of autodigestion. Fatty acid mobilisation results in increased ketone production.

3.109   AB

The principles of management of severe anaphylactic shock include: airway maintenance and oxygen; intravenous fluids to provide circulatory support; and subcutaneous or intramuscular adrenaline (epinephrine). Intravenous adrenaline may, in rare circumstances, be given, but at a much lower dose and only with ECG monitoring. Nebulised bronchodilators can help counteract the bronchospasm. Other drugs that might be helpful include aminophylline and hydrocortisone. Beta-blockers are contraindicated as they lower blood pressure and may cause bronchoconstriction.

3.110   ACE

Physiological and histological features of ARDS include: increased capillary permeability; interstitial and alveolar oedema; fibrin exudation; hyaline membrane formation; and, later, diffuse late interstitial and alveolar fibrosis.

3.111   BE

Perioperative myocardial ischaemia occurs most commonly in those with a history of a previous infarction, in the intraoperative period and on day 3 postoperatively. The more recent the MI, the greater the risk of re-infarction. Close intraoperative monitoring has been shown to reduce the risk of infarction in the higher-risk patient. The risk in patients without a cardiac history is < 1 in 70,000.

3.112   ACDF

Alpha-fetoprotein is secreted in high amounts by hepatocellular carcinomas and teratomas. It also occurs in some lung, gastric and pancreaticobiliary tumours. Medullary thyroid carcinoma is known to secrete calcitonin and is a reasonably good tumour marker. However, there are no known markers for parathyroid tumours. Acid phosphatase, but not alkaline phosphatase, is a tumour marker for prostate carcinoma. However, prostatic-specific antigen is a superior tumour marker for prostate carcinoma. Placental alkaline phosphatase is associated with some tumours but its lack of specificity means that it is not a clinically useful marker.

3.113   BG

Male sex, increased tumour thickness, the presence of ulceration, older age and mucosal involvement are predictors of a poor outcome in melanoma. The prognosis also depends on the lymph node involvement and growth pattern. The 5-year survival rate is 90% for stage I, 50% for stage II, 30% for stage III and < 1% for stage IV disease. While the so-called 'Celtic type' races appear more susceptible to the development of melanoma, non-white populations with melanoma have a worse overall outcome.

3.114   ABEF
Preconditions for a good screening test include:

* The disease must be an important health problem.
* There should be an accepted treatment.
* Facilities for diagnosis and treatment must be available.
* There should be a latent stage.
* The screening test should have both high sensitivity and specificity.
* The test should be acceptable to the population.
* The natural history of the disease should be adequately understood.
* There should be an agreed policy on which patients should be treated.
* Diagnosis and treatment should be relatively cost-effective.
* The screening should be an ongoing process.

For a screening test to be effective, early detection and treatment must lead to fewer deaths. An anaplastic carcinoma would carry such a poor prognosis that any screening test would make no difference to the outcome. Similarly, earlier detection of tumours with a short latent stage is unlikely to help.

3.115   BCEF
Hamartomas are not true tumours but represent overgrowth of one or more cell types that have normal constituents. However, they are arranged in irregular fashion (examples are haemangioma, lymphangioma, lipoma and neurofibroma). Sarcoma is a malignant tumour arising in tissues of mesenchymal origin. Sarcomas of soft tissue and bone are rare and represent < 1% of malignant neoplasms. A Krukenberg tumour is the name originally given to metastatic deposits on the ovaries secondary to a gastric tumour. In Zollinger–Ellison syndrome a gastrin-secreting pancreatic tumour is associated with peptic ulceration; > 50% are malignant. A high fasting serum gastrin level is diagnostic. Barrett's oesophagus is a metaplastic change from squamous to columnar epithelium in the distal oesophagus. It is premalignant condition.

3.116   AC
The development of lymph node metastases dramatically reduces survival. When regional lymph nodes are involved, the 5-year survival decreases to approximately 30%. Satellite lesions represent an aggressive tumour and microinvasion. Nodular melanomas are more aggressive than superficial spreading lesions. Other indicators of invasiveness include: vascular invasion; high mitotic rate; ulceration; and tumour-infiltrating lymphocytes.

3.117 ACD

Testicular tumours mostly spread to the para-aortic nodes, and not to the inguinal lymph nodes. Prostatic carcinoma characteristically produces metastases in the lumbar vertebrae as a result of the prostatic venous plexus drainage into the internal vertebral plexus. Prostatic tumours are adenocarcinomas with a variable degree of differentiation. This is reflected in their behaviour and the aggressiveness of their local and metastatic spread. Osteosarcoma preferentially spreads via blood to the lungs.

3.118 B

Beta-naphthylamine exposure has been strongly linked with bladder tumours. The human bladder mucosa secretes the enzyme β-glucuronidase, which splits β-naphthylamine and releases a carcinogen. Beta-naphthylamine is an aromatic amine and is a good example of remote carcinogenesis. The average latent period from exposure to disease development is 15 years. Other strong links with bladder carcinoma are benzidine exposure and smoking.

3.119 ABDE

Staging of malignant lesions for individual patients allows only a statistical risk of outcome for that patient. Accurate tumour staging cannot be made on the basis of a histological specimen alone, and requires additional information on nodal and distant disease. Pathological staging may be altered by the response to chemotherapy or irradiation treatment, and is known as 'downstaging'. Staging of tumours takes into account local tissue anatomy for individual primary tumour sites, including: invasion of tumours into the different layers of the wall of any viscus, and invasion into adjacent local structures.

3.120 AB

Bowen's disease is a skin disorder that may develop into squamous-cell carcinoma; histologically it is an intraepidermal carcinoma. It predominantly occurs on the legs. Keratoacanthoma is a benign self-involuting lesion, and molluscum contagiosum is an infective lesion. Basal-cell papillomas (seborrhoeic keratoses) are benign and have no malignant potential, as opposed to solar (actinic) keratoses, which do. A Spitz naevus is a variant of benign melanocytic lesions and can be mistaken histologically for malignant melanoma. It is most common in women under 30 years of age.

3.121   ABDE

Oncogenes are normal cell proteins that become abnormally activated in cancerous cells. They cause cells to proliferate through various mechanisms. Oncogenes and their corresponding oncoproteins are implicated when their encoded proteins become overexpressed, truncated, mutated or otherwise modified. The *erbB2* oncogene product, for example, is overexpressed in 20% of breast cancers. Oncogenes are also expressed during embryogenesis, regeneration and healing.

3.122   DEF

A tumour suppressor gene normally encodes products that inhibit growth and cell proliferation. It is a recessive gene and a mutation in one of the two copies of this gene will normally cause no harmful effect, as the remaining copy continues to code for a functional protein (Knudson hypothesis). Both copies must be affected before uncontrolled cellular growth and proliferation results.

Tumour suppressor genes were discovered as a result of studies in rare and inherited forms of cancer, particularly retinoblastoma. Retinoblastoma is the commonest malignant eye tumour of childhood. Most cases are diagnosed by the age of 3 years; 20–30% of cases affect both eyes. All of the bilateral cases and 15% of the unilateral cases are inherited as an autosomal dominant trait. The risk of retinoblastoma in the offspring of those with the genetic form of the disease is up to 50%.

TP53 is a tumour suppressor gene whose protein products cause cells to arrest in the G1 phase of the cell cycle. Mutations of this gene are common in cancers, occurring in up to 60% of instances (Li–Fraumeni syndrome; breast, gastric, lung and thyroid cancers). Other examples of tumour suppressor genes include *APC*, *hMSH2*, *hMLH1* and the *BRCA1* and *BRCA2* genes.

In contrast to tumour suppressor genes, oncogenes are deemed dominant as only one copy of the two genes needs to be affected for carcinogenesis. The oncogene v-*erbB2* is implicated in breast, ovarian, gastric and bladder carcinoma. The transcription factor *c-myc* is involved in Burkitt's lymphoma, small-cell lung cancer, multiple myeloma, testicular and prostate cancer; *c-myc* plays a role in gene amplification. It is found in normal cells but functions with less restriction in tumour cells.

K-*ras* is an oncogene implicated in colorectal, pancreatic and lung carcinomas as well as in leukaemia.

3.123   BDG

Alpha-fetoprotein is the fetal equivalent of plasma albumin and is produced by the fetal liver, yolk sac and intestine. It can be elevated in hepatocellular carcinoma (up to 90% of cases), testicular teratoma, pancreatic, biliary, gastric and bronchial cancers. Increased levels are also seen in hepatitis (viral). It is found in pregnancy, where high levels can be indicative of neural tube defects. A pure seminomatous germ-cell tumour does not produce α-fetoprotein.

3.124   BE

Malignant tumours have the potential to metastasise and therefore would include cholangiocarcinoma and adenocarcinoma. Adenocarcinoma tends to metastasise to the lymph nodes and liver. Cholangiocarcinoma spreads via lymphatics and the bloodstream. Adenomas are benign tumours but can undergo genetic mutations and progress to neoplasia. However, only 5% of colonic adenomas will progress to adenocarcinoma and malignancy. Similarly, only a minority of gallbladder adenomas will become malignant. Breast fibroadenoma does not have malignant potential. Basal-cell carcinoma is the commonest malignant skin tumour and is typically slow-growing and locally invasive. Metastases can occur, but are exceedingly rare.

3.125   ACEF

Bronchial carcinoma is the most common malignant tumour in the Western world, and is now the third most common cause of death in the UK. It carries the highest mortality of all malignancies in the UK and the USA. Bronchial carcinoma is usually advanced at the time of presentation. Normally, once there is mediastinal lymph node involvement, a curative resection cannot be performed. The UK incidence of lung cancer is decreasing in men, but increasing in women and is likely to reflect the altered smoking habits of contemporary women. Due to paraneoplastic syndromes, ectopic adrenocorticotrophic hormone (ACTH) may be produced, causing a fall in potassium, hyperglycaemia and an alkalosis. Similarly, SIADH can result in hyponatraemia. SIADH is commoner in small-cell cancers and is therefore associated with irresectability. Small-cell lung cancer is the most radiosensitive of all lung cancers.

3.126   CF

Radiotherapy is not the first-line treatment of oesophageal adenocarcinoma. Preoperative radiotherapy has conferred no advantage compared with surgery alone. In fact, adenocarcinomas are relatively resistant to radiotherapy. The primary treatment for gastric or rectal carcinoma is surgical resection. An adjuvant role for radiotherapy has been found by some studies of gastric cancer, particularly with regards to locoregional control. Radiotherapy is not, however, the primary mode of treatment of gastric cancer. Approximately 90% of oral and oropharyngeal tumours are squamous-cell carcinoma in origin, including those of the vocal folds. Early vocal fold tumours can be treated initially with radiotherapy. Advanced tumours may benefit from palliative radiotherapy.

Cystosarcoma phylloides tumour is a mixed connective tissue and epithelial tumour of the breast. It is fast-growing but only 15% are malignant. Treatment is local excision, but it may require chemo- or radiotherapy in metastatic cases. First-line treatment for anal cancer is now radiotherapy with or without chemotherapy, but most commonly the latter.

3.127   ABE

Familial adenomatous polyposis is an autosomal dominant premalignant condition (accounting for 1% of all colorectal carcinomas). Multiple polyps are found throughout the colon and rectum by the early teens. If left untreated, the polyps will become malignant. Paget's disease of the nipple is nearly always associated with an intraductal carcinoma in situ which, if left alone, will progress to invasive cancer. Acanthosis nigricans is a skin condition that is associated with malignancy, but is itself not a premalignant condition. Patients typically develop pruritic hyperkeratotic plaques affecting flexor surfaces such as the axilla. The tumours associated with acanthosis nigricans are mostly intra-abdominal, classically gastric carcinoma. Histologically, a keratoacanthoma resembles a squamous-cell carcinoma. However, it is not premalignant. Typically, keratoacanthomas grow rapidly but do not infiltrate beyond the sweat glands. After several weeks of such growth a keratoacanthoma regresses.

3.128   BEF

The programme was initiated in 1986 after the Forrest Report and screens women between 50 and 64 at 3-yearly intervals. There been no major increase in benign biopsies, but there has been an increase in the proportion of early-stage disease detected.

3.129 B
Experience from both the USA and the UK has shown that regular screening with Papanicolaou-stained (Pap) smears from the cervix can reduce mortality from cervical cancer. To date, studies on screening with regular chest radiographs or sputum cytology have shown no improved survival from lung cancer. Further trials are pending. There is no survival benefit for screening cancer of the ovary in the general population at present. However, there may be a strong case for screening a high-risk group with 'familial' ovarian cancer syndrome.

3.130 BCE
Malignant tumours are characterised by their invasiveness (an absolute criterion) and lack of ordered growth. They typically do not have a capsule. Malignant tumours contain cells with greater variation in size and shape, with increased cellular turnover and incomplete differentiation, than benign tumours. Loss of cellular adhesion at the tumour primary site is a major step in metastasis formation. Oncogene activation can occur in both benign and malignant tumours. Tumours > 2 mm^3 will require angiogenesis to sustain them. Since larger tumours are, in general, more likely to metastasise, the presence of angiogenesis may indicate malignancy.

3.131 AB
Alkylating agents are perhaps the oldest class of anti-cancer drug and are still in frequent use. Alkylating agents form covalent bonds in cellular DNA, thereby resulting in their de-activation. Mitomycin C, for example, is used in the treatment of gastric and bladder cancer. It is both an antibiotic and an alkylating agent. Vinca alkaloids are a separate class of chemotherapeutic agent and prevent spindle formation.

3.132 CD
Neuroblastoma is a tumour of the sympathetic nervous system, and is usually highly malignant. It mostly affects children and infants. Since neuroblastic tumours are derived from neural crest cells, they can affect the adrenal medulla (and adjacent retroperitoneal tissue), sympathetic neurones and melanocytes. Males and females are affected equally. Around 75% of neuroblastomas have metastasised at presentation. The presence of c-*myc* in tumour cells is associated with increased aggressiveness.

3.133 ABE

CEA is a water-soluble glycoprotein. It is elevated in less than 5% of patients with Dukes grade A colorectal cancer, 25% of Dukes B, 44% of Dukes C and approximately 65% of patients with distant metastases. It is not a useful diagnostic marker as it is increased in severe benign liver disease, inflammatory conditions (particularly of the gastrointestinal tract), trauma, infection, collagen diseases, renal impairment and smoking. It may assist in detecting tumour recurrence, especially in the liver following colorectal cancer resection. The half-life is 10 days.

3.134 ACE

Aromatic amines such as β-naphthylamine are associated with urinary tract (especially bladder) tumours in chemical workers who are particularly involved with dyes and pesticides. Painters, printers, mechanics and others working with petroleum derivatives and organic solvents (benzene exposure) are at an increased risk of developing leukaemia, lymphoma and multiple myeloma. Arsenic is used in pesticide manufacture and exposure also occurs in metal smelters. It is associated with skin and lung cancers as well as bladder tumours.

3.135 AD

Cancer registries obtain their data by identifying all death certificates that state 'cancer' as the cause of or contributing to death and then studying the notes of these patients. Postmortem findings contribute greatly to the accuracy of such data. Among other things, cancer registries can monitor the outcomes of ongoing treatment trials and compare current therapies and centres. In addition, they enable at-risk families to be identified for study and possibly screening. While they are a source of valuable local data, they are of particular value in providing a large information source for the collection of national data, thereby enabling national features and trends to be identified and studied and regional variations to be highlighted.

3.136   ACD

Hamartomas are benign overgrowths of fully differentiated normal components of the tissues in which they arise. In a hamartoma the proportion and composition of these normal tissue components differs greatly from the normal tissue structure. The most common hamartomas are vascular and include birthmarks such as port-wine stains. The polyps of Peutz–Jeghers syndrome are gastrointestinal hamartomas, while the associated lesion at the vermilion border of the lips is due to increased pigmentation. Although not neoplastic, hamartomas are mass lesions and, unlike true neoplasms, they cannot grow autonomously. Hamartomas require surgery if they cause obstruction, intussusception or bleeding. Hamartomas can take over a decade to double in size.

3.137   A

Adenomas are benign tumours of ductal or glandular epithelial cells. Consistent with their benign nature they are typically encapsulated and not invasive, although they can be premalignant. Nuclear pleomorphism is characteristic of malignancy, although some colorectal adenomas can display cellular characteristics intermediate between normality and malignancy. Adenomas can contain dysplastic cells. Annular lesions which grow in hollow organs and can cause stricturing are typically malignant. Neoplasms of squamous, columnar or transitional epithelial cells are papillomas if benign, or carcinomas if malignant. However, it is thought that there are no truly benign transitional-cell papillomas.

3.138   ABE

Oncogenes are normal cellular genes with the potential to cause malignant transformation when structurally and functionally mutated or abnormally or inappropriately expressed. They tend to code for proteins (oncoproteins) involved in key cellular regulatory processes. They can cause malignancy not only when their gene product is altered by mutation, but when they are over- or underexpressed or expressed at an inappropriate stage of the cell cycle. Because of the key regulatory roles of their products, oncogenes tend to be fundamental to cellular activity and hence highly conserved throughout evolution. Their discovery and much research work hinged on the discovery of tumour viruses containing viral analogues of these genes, derived from cellular oncogenes, which act as vectors for their transmission and for malignant transformation of host cells. The H-*ras* oncogene in the Harvey rat sarcoma virus is found in a variety of common human cancers.

3.139   ABC

Metastasis is facilitated by the ability of neoplastic cells to secrete angiogenic and angioproliferative factors to promote the development of new blood vessels and hence their own blood supply (as they grow beyond 1–2 mm). Tumour growth and metastasis both require angiogenesis. To metastasise, cells must overcome their normal cohesion and be able to invade the tissue, a property facilitated by the secretion of the enzyme protease. Cancer cells must adhere to the basement membrane to pass through. Adhesion to the basement membrane requires the expression of integrins (cell-surface receptors for basement-membrane components) but not cadherins, which enhance cell-to-cell adhesion.

3.140   D

In the cell cycle, the growth and proliferation of normal cells is regulated, and changes in the regulatory mechanisms may result in neoplastic transformation. Immediately following cell division, cells enter the G1 phase of high metabolic activity, but not DNA synthesis. DNA is synthesised in the next stage, the S stage. From there the cell enters the G2 stage, preparing for the M phase, or mitosis – which, as the DNA content of the cell is now double, results in the production of two diploid cells. All the stages, apart from G1, have fairly fixed durations and the growth rate of a tissue therefore depends on the length of time its cells spend in G1.

3.141   BCDF

Combination chemotherapy is used to combat drug resistance. Combinations of drugs have at least as much toxicity, if not more, than single agents. Many chemotherapy agents, such as doxorubicin and vinca alkaloids, are metabolised in the liver so toxicity would be increased in liver impairment. Highly emetogenic drugs require treatment with the serotonin antagonists (5-HT$_3$) such as granisetron. Bone marrow suppression may present as bleeding, such as epistaxis. Hair loss from chemotherapy is almost always reversible after the course of treatment, even if the quality of regrowth may be altered. Creatinine clearance is a measure of renal function. Drugs excreted by the kidneys are therefore removed more rapidly when renal function is good.

3.142   ACDEF
The early complications of radiotherapy reflect the sensitivity of rapidly growing cells to radiation damage. They include desquamation lesions of the skin and gastrointestinal tract (inflammation, bleeding and ulceration), infertility and bone marrow suppression, which can lead to bone marrow failure. Hypothyroidism is a late complication of exposure of the thyroid gland to radiation, and may also complicate radio-iodine treatment for thyroid malignancy. The production of secondary malignancies is now recognised as a late complication of radiotherapy and may develop from 3 years after therapy.

3.143   BEFG
Bromocriptine inhibits prolactin secretion and is used to suppress lactation in the treatment of galactorrhoea. Cimetidine is an H_2-antagonist used in dyspepsia. It interferes with cytochrome P450 in the liver and this leads to raised oestrogen levels sufficient to cause gynaecomastia. This is a dose-dependent side effect. Similarly, liver disease can cause oestrogen/androgen imbalance and gynaecomastia. Oral corticosteroids cause a redistribution of fat and Cushing's syndrome, but they do not lead to gynaecomastia. Pituitary tumours and hyperthyroidism may cause gynaecomastia. Around 10% of testicular tumours (usually teratomas) are associated with gynaecomastia.

3.144   ACDE
BXO is a dyskeratotic skin disorder affecting the prepuce, glans or urethral meatus. Similarly to condyloma, erythroplasia of Queyrat and Bowen's disease, BXO is considered precancerous. Paget's disease of the breast is associated with an underlying breast malignancy and is not premalignant. Both Peutz–Jeghers syndrome and familial adenomatous polyposis predispose to malignancies in the bowel. Severe metaplasia in a Barrett's oesophagus may also progress to oesophageal adenocarcinoma, the increased risk being approximately 20-fold.

3.145 ADE
Results of screening programmes for cancer are limited by selection, length and lead-time bias. Selection bias arises from the tendency of people who enrol on screening programmes to be more health-conscious and are therefore atypical of the general population. Length bias is the tendency for screening to detect a disproportionate number of cancers which are slow-growing and have a better prognosis anyway. Lead-time bias occurs when screening advances the date at which diagnosis is made. This, therefore, lengthens the calculated survival time without necessarily altering the date of death.

3.146 ACDF
Potentially premalignant lesions of the oesophagus include: Plummer–Vinson syndrome (oesophageal web); corrosive oesophagitis; achalasia; Barrett's oesophagus; and scleroderma involvement of the oesophagus. There is a 20-fold increased risk of developing oesophageal cancer in Barrett's oesophagus. There is an increased risk of oesophageal cancer with achalasia and with hiatus hernia.

3.147 ACE
Bladder, cervical and laryngeal cancer are all smoking-related. No known association exists for the leukaemias and lymphomas.

3.148 ACEFGH
Deaths reportable to the coroner include: dead on arrival; deaths within 24 hours of emergency admission to hospital; deaths during or within 24 hours of an operation/anaesthetic/invasive procedure; deaths occurring as a result of an accident; unnatural, criminal or suspicious deaths, including those caused by neglect, suicide or abuse; and deaths from poisoning, drugs or acute or chronic alcohol abuse. Industrial or occupational diseases leading to death, as well as deaths from medical or surgical mishap should also be reported. Also reportable are: the death of a prisoner while in hospital; stillbirths; cases of hypothermia leading to death; deaths in public places, fires, police custody or prison; deaths where a property has been broken into; and deaths where the police are involved. Notifiable diseases have to be reported to the Consultant in Communicable Disease Control (CCDC). At present, the reporting of AIDS to the CCDC is voluntary.

3.149 All true

People require sufficient information before deciding to give their consent to a procedure, and therefore all the treatment options should be listed and explained. If someone is not offered sufficient information as reasonably needed to make a decision (and in an understandable form), then consent may not be valid.

3.150 ADE

DIC is a multisystem disorder characterised by simultaneous activation of the coagulation and fibrinolytic pathways. Common causes include sepsis, malignancy (especially adenocarcinoma), trauma and obstetric emergencies (placenta abruption, amniotic fluid embolism). Although DIC usually manifests as bleeding, some patients display thrombosis. Progressive consumption of all the coagulation factors and platelets leads to a characteristic laboratory profile of prolongation of the prothrombin time (PT), activated partial thrombin time (APTT) and thrombin time (TT) and falling fibrinogen and platelets. Increased fibrinolysis is indicated by rising concentrations of fibrinogen degradation products or D-dimers. Although similar findings may be seen in hepatic insufficiency, DIC may be diagnosed by demonstrating deteriorating coagulation abnormalities in conjunction with a likely clinical cause. The mainstay of care is treatment of the underlying cause, replacement of the deficient factors with fresh-frozen plasma, cryoprecipitate and platelets.

3.151 BDE

The essential components of TPN are nitrogen, carbohydrate, fat, minerals (calcium, magnesium, iron, zinc, manganese, copper, fluoride, iodine, chloride) and vitamins.

3.152 All true

Central venous line insertion may cause trauma to adjacent tissues with consequent haemorrhage and pneumothorax. If it is left open then air may enter the blood, causing venous air embolism. Systemic arterial air embolism may occur if the cannula is mistakenly placed in the carotid artery.

3.153 ABCF
Tumour markers are substances that are present in the body at a concentration proportional to the tumour burden. They are not always tumour-specific – for example, human chorionic gonadotrophin levels may be elevated in pregnancy, germ-cell tumours and gestational trophoblastic disease. Tumour markers are most commonly used to monitor therapeutic responses. However, they may also aid in diagnosis, have a role in the detection of relapse and provide prognostic information. For example, in the case of testicular germ-cell tumours, the level of tumour markers before treatment is an important predictor of outcome. CA-125 has not been detected in the normal ovary, but PSA is found in the normal prostate.

3.154 BDE
The absolute criterion for malignancy is invasiveness. Malignant tumours exhibit cells with greater variation in size and shape than benign tumours. There is increased cellular turnover and incomplete differentiation.

3.155 AC
Thrombophlebitis migrans is a condition causing recurrent thrombotic episodes in the superficial and deep veins, especially of the extremities. Many cases are idiopathic (or form a part of Buerger's disease) and show a diffuse inflammatory action. Thrombophlebitis migrans is also a well-known complication of a deep-seated cancer, the usual sites of primary tumour being the pancreas (tail and body), lung, stomach and female genital tract.

3.156 AD
Hepatitis A is an RNA virus and hepatitis B a DNA virus. The incubation period of hepatitis A is between 2 and 3 weeks. Hepatitis A accounts for 20–40% of all cases of viral hepatitis. It affects children and young adults particularly. It rarely causes fulminant hepatitis and does not give rise to a carrier state.

3.157 ABE
Numerous organisms can cause infection and abdominal pain in HIV-infected individuals. The well-documented organisms include: crypto-sporidia; cytomegaloviruses; *Mycobacterium tuberculosis*; *Salmonella*, *Shigella* and *Campylobacter* spp.; *Neisseria gonorrhoeae*; *Treponema pallidum*; *Mycobacterium avium-intracellulare*; *Listeria monocytogenes*; *Entamoeba histolytica*; *Giardia lamblia*; *Isospora belli*; *Candida albicans*; *Histoplasma* spp.; and herpes simplex virus. Kaposi's sarcoma is a vascular tumour.

3.158 ACF
Streptococcus pyogenes is β-haemolytic and belongs to Lancefield group A. Staphylococci are found in clusters; streptococci are found in pairs or chains. *Streptococcus* spp. produce streptolysins O and S, hyaluronidase, streptokinase, leukocidin and an erythrogenic toxin that causes scarlet fever. It is associated with rheumatic fever, carditis and glomerulonephritis as immunological sequelae. It is sensitive to penicillins.

3.159 CDE
The predominant commensal bacteria of the skin is *Staphylococcus epidermidis*. Others include *Staphylococcus aureus*, micrococci, coryneforms and anaerobic cocci. The lower respiratory tract is usually sterile. The predominant bacterial flora of the oropharynx are *Streptococcus viridans*, coryneforms and *Neisseria* spp. Many anaerobic bacteria colonise the colon, especially *Bacteroides fragilis*. The other main groups of commensal skin bacteria include members of the genus *Clostridia*. Aerobic bacteria such as *Escherichia coli* and *Enterococcus* spp. are also present in large numbers. Lactobacilli are the predominant species in the vagina. Others include *Gardnerella vaginalis* and anaerobes.

3.160 ADE
Phagocytosis is the process whereby cells – such as neutrophils and macrophages – ingest solid particles (involving adhesion of the target to the cell surface), facilitated by opsonisation. These cells fuse to form a phagosome, which further fuses with lysosomes, leading to the formation of a phagolysosome. It is within these that intracellular killing of micro-organisms occurs. The neutrophils produce microbicidal agents which act dependently or independently of oxygen. In oxygen-dependent mechanisms neutrophils produce hydrogen peroxide, peroxide anions, hydroxyl radicals and singlet oxygen. The oxygen-independent mechanisms involve lysozyme (muramidase), lactoferrin (which chelates iron and is required for bacterial growth), cationic protein formation and low pH inside phagocytic vacuoles. Release of lysosomal products from the cell damages local tissue by proteolysis via enzymes such as elastase and collagenase, activates coagulation factor XII, and attracts other leucocytes into the area. Some of the compounds released increase vascular permeability, while others are pyrogens, producing systemic fever by acting on the hypothalamus.

3.161   BDE
Intravascular haemolysis may result from the mechanical destruction of red cells by prosthetic heart valves or arterial grafts, in arteriovenous malformations or after severe physical exercise. Immune-mediated intravascular haemolysis is only usually encountered in the potent antibody–antigen interactions seen following ABO-mismatched transfusion. Most autoimmune haemolytic anaemias produce red cell destruction in the reticuloendothelial system. DIC may cause microangiopathic haemolysis with red cell destruction in the microcirculation.

3.162   ABCE
If oxygen delivery to the brain is reduced, agitation and coma can occur. Blood pressure may still be normal in compensated shock. Reduced renal perfusion and compensatory mechanisms attempt to preserve vascular volume and urine output will fall. In a hypovolaemic state, peripheral vascular resistance is decreased to preserve flow to vital organs. The normal response to hypovolaemic shock is tachycardia; however, with progression, bradycardia and even cardiac arrest may occur.

3.163   BDEFGH
Haemorrhage and septicaemia cause a low CVP and low blood pressure. A high CVP is caused by any factor that impedes venous return to the heart or reduces the output from the right ventricle. This in turn leads to low cardiac output and so low blood pressure.

3.164   BDE
Hyperphosphataemia and hypocalcaemia may be seen in chronic renal failure. Stress ulceration is associated with ARF and may be prevented by sucralfate (cytoprotection and pepsin adsorption). Renal hypoperfusion is associated with avid sodium retention with minimal excretion into the urine (< 20 mmol/l). Indications for renal biopsy include: unclear pathogenesis; suspicion of glomerular disease or interstitial nephritis; or prolonged (4–6 weeks) renal failure.

3.165   ACDE
The catabolic phase of the metabolic response to injury is accompanied by increased energy expenditure and a negative nitrogen balance. The size and duration of the response are directly related to the severity of the trauma or surgical insult.

3.166 ADE

A meningioma is a benign tumour of the meninges. A rhabdomyoma is a benign tumour of striated muscle (its malignant counterpart is a rhabdomyosarcoma). A chondrosarcoma is a malignant tumour of cartilage.

3.167 D

Metastasis is the spread of a tumour from one part of the body to another that is not directly interconnected. A variety of factors play a role: loss of cellular cohesion and cytoarchitecture, initiation of angiogenesis and adhesion molecules. Transluminal metastases are uncommon. Basal-cell carcinomas invade locally and metastases are rare. Osteosarcoma typically spreads via the bloodstream, most commonly to the lungs. It can also spread to other bones. The extensive venous plexus surrounding the prostate makes haematogenous spread likely. Lymphatic drainage nodes generally follow the path of arteries.

3.168 ABEFG

Hypercalcaemia may be part of a paraneoplastic syndrome of numerous malignancies, including carcinoma of the bronchus. Bone lysis occurs in multiple myeloma, giving rise to hypercalcaemia. Hypoparathyroidism reduces serum calcium, whereas hyperparathyroidism raises it (as does hyperthyroidism). Renal failure can lead to secondary hyper-parathyroidism, so raising serum calcium levels. Citrate used in the storage of blood binds ionised calcium and so reduces the serum level.

3.169 ABDE

Squamous-cell carcinomas are the second most common cutaneous malignancy. They are also known as epidermoid carcinomas or epitheliomas. Sun damage is a major risk factor, resulting in carcinoma in situ, followed by an invasive carcinoma.

A Merkel-cell carcinoma (also known as trabecular carcinoma) is a rare but highly aggressive tumour derived from the Merkel-cell population, which are primitive neuroendocrine (APUD) cells in the skin. These tumours occur mostly in elderly people. They tend to occur on sun-exposed sites, particularly the head, neck and limbs. The prognosis is poor, with local recurrence developing in 40% of cases and nodal metastases in up to 65%. Approximately half the patients are dead within 2 years.

A dermatofibroma is a red or brown small papule or nodule containing fibroblastic tissue, usually found on the legs and with no known aetiology or malignant potential.

Bowen's disease is a skin disorder that may develop into squamous-cell carcinoma; histologically it is an intraepidermal carcinoma. It predominantly occurs on the legs. Bowen's disease of the glans of the penis is called 'erythroplasia of Queyrat'.

A solar (actinic) keratosis is a potentially precancerous condition, frequently seen on the head and face, typically in sun-exposed older people. Treatment can be by excision, cryotherapy or the use of 5-FU cream.

3.170   ACE
Tourniquets, even when used in an appropriate manner, will lead to vascular damage and thrombosis, soft-tissue injury and nerve injury. It is important to record the time when the tourniquet is inflated. It should not remain constantly inflated for more than 2 hours. It is good practice to release the tourniquet before suturing the wound in order to identify the bleeding vessels and so prevent postoperative haemorrhage. (An opposite point of view states that once the tourniquet is released the reactive hyperaemia in the limb leads to significant blood loss from a multitude of small vessels – this is mainly an orthopaedic point of view and it is good practice for surgical trainees to consider releasing the tourniquet before closure.) The tourniquet pressure should be just above arterial pressure – otherwise bleeding would obscure the operating field. A tourniquet must be used as part of the Bier's block technique; if it is not, toxic levels of local anaesthetic would reach into the general circulation.

3.171   ABC
A fracture haematoma aids fracture healing by sealing off the fracture site and providing a framework for the influx of inflammatory cells and fibroblasts. Factors such as FGF and PDGF, which are released by inflammatory cells, stimulate osteoprogenitor cells to differentiate into osteoblasts and osteoclasts. The histology of healing bone shows disorganised elements of bone formation and destruction (osteoblastic and osteoclastic activity) and has a similar picture to that in an osteosarcoma. It usually takes a minimum of 3 weeks for calcified tissue (callus) to be seen on X-ray in an adult. Reduced callus formation occurs when fracture movement is minimised, for example by internal fixation.

3.172 BCDE

Infection is an early complication of fractures, especially when open. Ideally, open fractures should be fixed within 4–6 hours of injury. All patients with open fractures should be given antibiotics. Volkmann's ischaemic contracture occurs following an arterial injury or compartment syndrome where muscle is replaced by inelastic fibrous tissue. This may lead to claw hand or toes. Tendon rupture is a well-recognised late complication of fractures. Extensor pollicis longus rupture occurs (6–12 weeks) after fracture of the lower radius, and the long head of biceps may rupture following a humeral-neck fracture. Myositis ossificans is a form of heterotopic calcification occurring in soft tissue, notably after dislocation of the elbow or a blow to the brachialis, deltoid or quadriceps muscles. Treatment includes initial rest, then gentle active movements. Occasionally, excision of the bony mass is required. Algodystrophy (Sudek's atrophy) is characterised by a painful post-traumatic extremity. Late trophic changes are seen, with features of patchy osteoporosis on X-ray.

3.173 ABDE

Non-union is caused by: unrecognised delayed union; wide distraction and separation of the fracture surfaces; soft-tissue interposition; excessive movement at the fracture site; or poor local blood supply. Painless movement at the fracture site is diagnostic of non-union, as distinct from delayed union, which is painful. Two types of non-union are described: hypertrophic (bulbous bone-ends) and atrophic (no calcification at bone-ends). Non-union is occasionally symptomless, needing no treatment. Management includes functional bracing, electrical stimulation, which may promote osteogenesis, and internal or external fixation. Bone grafts are required for atrophic non-union.

3.174 BCE

Causes of delayed union include an inadequate blood supply, infection, incorrect immobilisation and an intact fellow bone (such as the fibula in a tibial fracture). The fracture site is usually tender and the fracture remains visible, with very little callus formation, periosteal reaction or sclerosis at the bone-ends. Continued treatment is required and includes functional bracing, an excellent method of promoting bony union. A fracture should undergo internal fixation and bone grafting if union is delayed for more than 6 months and in the absence of any callus formation.

3.175   BCDF

Paget's disease of bone is characterised by enlargement and thickening of the bone but the internal architecture is abnormal and the bone is unusually brittle. It affects men and women equally, most commonly from the age of 50 years. The most commonly affected sites are the pelvis and tibia. An elevated alkaline phosphatase indicates increased osteoblastic activity. Complications include nerve compression, fractures, osteoarthritis, osteosarcoma, high-output cardiac failure and hypercalcaemia. Treatment focuses on suppressing bone turnover and includes the use of calcitonin and bisphosphonates. Surgery may be required for pathological fractures and nerve entrapment states.

3.176   AC

Osteomyelitis may occur after any operation on bone, but especially after implantation of foreign material, such as prostheses. The organisms may come from the theatre environment, patient, surgeon or indirectly from a distant focus. It may present early (within 3 months) or late. The organisms are usually a mixture of pathogenic bacteria (*Staphylococcus aureus*, *Proteus* spp., *Pseudomonas* spp.). Predisposing factors include soft-tissue damage, bone death, poor contact between implant and bone, loosening and corrosion of the implant. Elimination of any focus of infection, optimal intraoperative sterility, prophylactic antibiotics, close fit and secure fixation of the implant will reduce the risk of postoperative osteomyelitis. MRI is not helpful in the early infection as it cannot distinguish between infection and normal postoperative changes. However, it may demonstrate collections of pus in late infections.

3.177   AD

Avascular necrosis occurs following an interruption of the arterial blood supply to a bone or following intra- or extraosseus venous insufficiency. Susceptible bones include the femoral and humeral heads, femoral condyles, capitum (when avulsed), proximal pole of the scaphoid, lunate and talus. The blood supply to the femoral head arises from the joint capsule. The femoral head is susceptible after an intracapsular (subcapital) but not an extracapsular (intertrochanteric) fracture.

3.178 BCDE

Acute osteomyelitis is most often found in children. In adults it is associated with immunosuppression and diabetes. The organism is most commonly *Staphylococcus aureus*. Others include *Streptococcus pyogenes* and *S. pneumoniae*. In children under 4 years, *Haemophilus influenzae* is fairly common. Patients with sickle cell disease are more prone to *Salmonella* infection. Organisms settle in the metaphysis, most often at the proximal end of the femur. In adults, the thoracolumbar spine is the most common site for haematogenous infection. X-ray changes (lytic or sclerotic changes, periosteal reaction) usually take 10 days to 2 weeks to become apparent. The first X-ray change seen is that of soft-tissue swelling.

3.179 ACD

Lymphoedema is an accumulation of tissue fluid as a result of a defect in the lymphatic system, principally affecting the legs (80%). However, it may be found in the arm, face and genitalia. Lymphoedema may be divided into primary (familial) and secondary. Secondary lymphoedema in Western countries is usually the result of surgical excision or radiotherapy to lymph nodes. On a worldwide scale, infection is much more common. The worm *Wuchereria bancrofti* causes filiariasis which leads to lymphoedema.

3.180 CDE

'Coralline clot' is a fine granular coral-like mass of platelets deposited on the endothelium, and is otherwise known as 'white thrombus'. 'Propagative clot' is red, slippery, non-adherent, and particularly likely to break up and form emboli. It is also known as 'red thrombus'. Aspirin, not anticoagulants, has an effect on platelet aggregation.

3.181 BD

Of all branchial cysts, 60% ooccur in men. Although the highest incidence is found in the third decade, they may occur between 1 and 70 years of age. Two-thirds are found on the left, and 2% are bilateral. Two-thirds of branchial cysts are anterior to sternocleidomastoid in the upper third of the neck. The most common presenting features are continuous or intermittent swelling or pain. Infection only occurs in 15% of cases. The cysts are lined by stratified squamous epithelium. Branchial cysts contain straw-coloured fluid in which cholesterol crystals can be found.

3.182   ABE
Of all salivary gland adenomas, 80% arise in the parotid gland. Around 80% are pleomorphic adenomas and 80% arise in the superficial lobe. Most adenomas present in middle age or later in life, and they have an equal sex incidence. Parotid adenomas usually occur in the superficial part of the gland, external to the plane of the lower branches of the facial nerve. Occasionally they occur in the deep part of the gland. A parotid adenoma is a benign tumour and does not impinge on the nerves to cause a facial palsy. Frey's syndrome is a late complication of parotidectomy, occurring in as many as 25% of patients. It results from the division of the parasympathetic secretory motor fibres originally innervating the gland. These nerve fibres regenerate in the skin where they assume control of sweat gland activity. Facial sweating then occurs in response to salivatory stimuli (gustatory sweating).

3.183   ABD
Of all parotid tumours, 80% are benign and 80% of these are pleomorphic adenomas. Around 15% of salivary gland neoplasms are found in the submandibular gland. A proportion of tumours are slow-growing, but should not be biopsied as they are at risk of tumour-seeding along the tract. Otalgia (referred pain) may be a presenting feature.

3.184   ADE
There are numerous causes of raised serum calcium levels. The most common include metastatic bony tumour deposits, primary hyper-parathyroidism and multiple myeloma. Secondary hyperparathyroidism occurs in response to a low serum calcium level. Tertiary hyper-parathyroidism is most commonly seen in chronic renal failure. Other causes of hypercalcaemia include thyrotoxicosis, Paget's disease of bone, sarcoidosis, vitamin D intoxication, Addison's disease, thiazide diuretics, tuberculosis and familial hypocalciuric hypercalcaemia.

3.185   ACD
Most patients who undergo a gastrectomy fail to regain their preoperative weight. Low serum calcium, vitamin C and iron levels (but not frank deficiency) are seen, as the hypochlorhydria interferes with their absorption. Vitamin B_{12} deficiency develops due to diminished levels of intrinsic factor from the stomach. This may be corrected by injections of hydroxocobalamin every 3 months.

3.186   AB

Rectal bleeding is the most common initial symptom (45% of cases); 30% of patients complain of pain or sensation of a mass. The human papillomavirus (usually type 16) may cause intraepithelial neoplasia, which with time progresses to anal carcinoma. This virus is found in approximately 70% of patients. Other risk factors for anal carcinoma include a history of cervical or vaginal cancer, history of sexually transmitted disease and immunosuppression following solid organ transplantation. Lymphatic drainage – above the dentate line, flows to the perirectal and paravertebral nodes; below the dentate line, drainage is through the inguinal and femoral nodes. Anal carcinoma is relatively radiosensitive. Presently, combination radiotherapy and chemotherapy (5-FU ± mitomycin or 5-FU + cisplatin) is used as initial standard first-line treatment. Abdominoperineal resection is reserved for recurrent or resistant tumours.

3.187   ABCE

Crohn's disease is a granulomatous inflammatory disorder involving the whole thickness of the bowel wall (any part of the gastrointestinal tract from mouth to anus). UC is a non-granuloma process that only involves the mucosa. This difference may explain the higher incidence of stricture, obstruction and fistula formation in Crohn's disease. UC invariably involves the rectum and extends proximally towards the caecum, and can sometimes cause a 'backwash ileitis'. Perianal problems (fissures, fistulae, skin tags) are much more commonly seen in Crohn's disease than in UC.

3.188   CDE

Horseshoe kidney is more common in men. The anatomical location and blood supply is very variable. They are more prone to infection and calculi formation due to relative upper-tract stasis. They are also more prone to trauma.

3.189   All true

The causes of neuropathic bladder dysfunction can be divided into cerebral lesions (CVA, dementia, parkinsonism), spinal lesions (trauma, multiple sclerosis, spina bifida), and peripheral nerve lesions (following pelvic surgery or diabetes mellitus). Lesions of the sacral cord or peripheral nerves cause an underactive detrusor and urethra. Lesions of the supraspinal cord cause loss of inhibitory impulses, so causing detrusor over-reactivity and uncoordinated activity of detrusor and urethra. Lesions above the pons cause loss of cerebral inhibition and may produce an overactive detrusor. Detrusor and urethral activity remain uncoordinated.

3.190   AC
Staghorn calculi (also known as 'struvite') are composed of magnesium, ammonium and phosphate. They form when urine pH > 7. They are associated with *Proteus* spp. and other Gram-negative organisms that contain the enzyme urease. This results in the splitting of urea into ammonium ions, so alkalinising the urine.

3.191   CD
Osteosarcoma is most commonly found at the metaphyses of long bones, and usually presents in the second and third decades of life. It is a rare but well-recognised complication of Paget's disease and this accounts for the second peak in incidence around the sixth decade. Osteosarcomas may be osteolytic, osteoblastic or show a mixed picture on X-ray. Sun-ray spicules represent new bone formation once the cortex has been destroyed. Bone formation in Codman's triangle is due to elevation of the periosteum by invasion of tumour through the cortex.

3.192   ACDE
The most common causes of conductive deafness include wax, acute otitis media, secretory otitis media, chronic otitis media, barotrauma, otosclerosis, injuries to the tympanic membrane and otitis externa. Less common causes include tumours of the middle ear and traumatic ossicular dislocation. Sensorineural deafness has a number of causes, including infections such as mumps, herpes zoster, meningitis and syphilis. Other causes of senorineural deafness include congenital– maternal rubella, cytomegalovirus, toxoplasmosis, prolonged exposure to loud noises, drugs (aspirin, aminoglycosides), Ménière's disease, head injury and acoustic neuroma. Metabolic causes of sensorineural deafness include diabetes and hypothyroidism. In Paget's disease there may be a mixed hearing loss, with conduction and sensorineural deafness. This may be due to ankylosis of the stapes, or compression on the VIIIth cranial nerve in the auditory foramen by bone.

3.193   CDG
Meckel's diverticulum occurs in 2% of the population and affects men twice as often as women. It is classically found 0.6 m from the ileocaecal valve on the antimesenteric border of the small intestine and is approximately 5 cm long. It is a true diverticulum with a mucous membrane and a muscular coat and may be connected to the umbilicus by either a fibrous band or a complete fistula – remnants of the vitellointestinal duct. Most cases of Meckel's diverticulum are asymptomatic, but 20% contain heterotopic gastric or pancreatic mucosa. Complications of Meckel's diverticulum include diverticulitis, intussusception, ulceration and gastrointestinal bleeding, intestinal obstruction and perforation. If a Meckel's diverticulum is found incidentally, it should be left alone, especially if it is non-inflamed with a wide neck.

3.194   CDE
Amyloidosis is a disorder in which extracellular proteinaceous substances (protein fibrils) are deposited in body tissues, locally or systemically. Amyloidosis may be of primary or secondary aetiology, and is linked with chronic disease conditions that are usually inflammatory (rheumatoid arthritis, Crohn's disease) or caused by infections (tuberculosis); it is also associated with multiple myeloma, Hodgkin's disease and Waldenström's macroglobulinaemia. Other forms of amyloidosis are familial and isolated (as in Alzheimer's disease).

3.195   BCDE
Postsplenectomy sepsis can present 20 years after splenectomy and carries a high mortality (50%). It is prevented by penicillin prophylaxis, which should be lifelong. The micro-organisms most likely to lead to infection include *Pneumococcus* and *Meningococcus* spp. and *H. influenzae*. Other infections include those due to *Escherichia coli* and malaria.

3.196   BDE
Long-standing massive splenomegaly is known to be caused by chronic malaria, chronic myeloid leukaemia, myelofibrosis, kala-azar and schistosomiasis. Chagas' disease causes oesophageal and gastrointestinal dilation. Hepatitis C is associated with cirrhosis of the liver, which may in turn produce splenomegaly. However, the splenomegaly is only moderate.

3.197   AFG

Keloid scars are more common on pigmented skin, burns and trauma wounds and in those with a past history of keloid scars. There is excessive production and contraction of fibrous tissue. Greater success has been claimed for triamcinolone (steroid) injections which produce collagen lysis, whereas surgical excision may only result in a larger scar. Keloids occur on the dorsal areas of the body and over the face and deltopectoral region. The difference between keloid scarring and hypertrophic scarring is that the former heals by extending beyond the original boundary of incision, whereas the latter is a thickened scar within the initial incision.

3.198   ABC

Circumcision in infancy is associated with an extremely low risk of developing penile cancer in adult life. There is no proved association between prostatic cancer and vasectomy.

3.199   BD

Secondary haemorrhage occurs 5–10 days postoperatively. It is due to local sepsis, dislodgement of clot/sloughing or ligature erosion. This phenomenon is commonly seen in patients undergoing transurethral resection of the prostate (TURP). Anticoagulation may cause bleeding problems, but these are not classified as secondary haemorrhage.

3.200   BC

A reduced serum calcium level causes an increase in PTH release. PTH increases the serum calcium level by acting on the kidney, bone and gut (indirectly). It causes increased renal reabsorption of calcium and increased conversion of vitamin D to 1,25-DHCC. In turn, 1,25-DHCC stimulates the intestinal absorption of calcium. Osteoclasts are also activated to increase bone resorption and so raise calcium levels.

3.201 ADE

ARDS is an acute, diffuse inflammatory process resulting from direct or indirect pulmonary injury. It is most commonly seen in sepsis but can also occur after trauma, burns, inhalation injuries, shock and pancreatitis. In postoperative surgical patients, abdominal sepsis or central line sepsis should be considered. Indirect or direct lung injury initiates an abnormal behaviour and movement of neutrophils, platelets and macrophages. Neutrophils and platelets attach to capillary endothelium causing capillary leak. This leads to oedema of lung tissue and movement of neutrophils and erythrocytes into the lung parenchyma. Lung lymph flow is increased and there is thickening of the alveolar–capillary membrane. This results in impaired oxygen diffusion and reduced lung compliance as the alveolus is surrounded by fluid. In addition, some of the fluid in the pulmonary parenchyma may leak into the alveoli, giving the characteristic appearance of a hyaline membrane.

ARDS is characterised by refractory hypoxemia (PaO_2 < 8 kPa at FIO_2 > 0.4), alveolar inflammation and oedema, reduced total compliance (< 30 ml/cmH$_2$O) and a PaO_2 (in mmHg) to FIO_2 ratio of < 200 (normal is approximately 500). Pulmonary fibrosis in the later stages of the disease leads to a decrease in the functional residual capacity, further decrease in lung compliance, and an increase in the shunt effect. Pulmonary signs are often minimal or non-specific, the patient simply being breathless, progressively tachypnoeic, hypoxic and then cyanotic. Chest X-ray may be normal in the early stages but later shows bilateral diffuse pulmonary infiltration. Treatment, in addition to eliminating the precipitating cause, involves ventilating the patient in an Intensive Care Unit. Patients are usually nursed in the prone position. The tidal volume should be kept low (approximately 6 ml/kg) and so should the pulmonary capillary wedge pressure (high pressures exacerbate pulmonary oedema). The mortality of this condition is as high as 50–70%.

INDEX

Note to reader: Entries are indexed by question number, not by page number.

Index

Index

Index

Index

PASTEST

PasTest has been established since 1972 and is the leading provider of exam-related medical revision courses and books in the UK. The company has a dedicated customer services team to ensure that doctors can easily get up to date information about our products and to ensure that their orders are dealt with efficiently. Our extensive experience means that we are always one step ahead when it comes to knowledge of the current trends and contents of the Royal College exams.

PasTest revision books have helped thousands of candidates prepare for their exams. These may be purchased through bookshops, over the telephone or online at our website. All books are reviewed prior to publication to ensure that they mirror the needs of candidates and therefore act as an invaluable aid to exam preparation.

100% Money Back Guarantee
We're sure you will find our study books invaluable, but in the unlikely event that you are not entirely happy, we will give you your money back – guaranteed.

Delivery to your Door
With a busy lifestyle, nobody enjoys walking to the shops for something that may or may not be in stock. Let us take the hassle and deliver direct to your door. We will despatch your book within 24 hours of receiving your order. We also offer free delivery on books for medical students to UK addresses.

How to Order
www.pastest.co.uk
To order books safely and securely online, shop at our website.

Telephone: +44 (0)1565 752000
Have your credit card to hand when you call.
Fax: +44 (0) 1565 650264
Fax your order with your debit or credit card details.

PasTest Ltd, FREEPOST, Knutsford, Cheshire WA16 7BR
Send your order with your cheque (made payable to PasTest Ltd) or debit /credit card details to the above address. (Please complete your address details on the reverse of the cheque.)

PASTEST REVISION BOOKS FOR MRCS

Look out for this book's sister title

Intercollegiate MRCS: Clinical Problem Solving Vol 1
C L H Chan   ISBN: 1 904627 23 4
This book is written specifically for the new intercollegiate examination and contains Extended Matching Questions with complete explanations for every question.

Also Available from PasTest for Intercollegiate MRCS revision:

Essential Lists for the Intercollegiate MRCS
M Murphy   ISBN: 1 901 198 23 5

Viva Practice for MRCS (Part 3)
C L H Chan   ISBN: 1 904 627 19 6

Surgical Short Cases for the MRCS Clinical Examination
C Parchment Smith   ISBN: 1 901 198 44 8

To order any of the above titles, please contact PasTest on:
01565 752000
PasTest Ltd, FREEPOST, Knutsford, Cheshire, WA16 7BR
Fax: 01565 650264; E-mail: books@pastest.co.uk
Or order online at www.pastest.co.uk

PASTEST COURSES

PASTEST: the key to exam success, the key to your future

PasTest is dedicated to helping doctors to pass their professional examinations. We have 30 years of specialist experience in medical education and over 3000 doctors attend our revision courses each year.

Experienced lecturers:
Many of our lecturers are also examiners and teach in a lively and interesting way in order to:
* reflect current trends in exams
* give plenty of mock exam practice
* provide valuable advice on exam technique

Outstanding accelerated learning:
Our up-to-date and relevant course material includes MCQs, colour slides, X-rays, ECGs, EEGs, clinical cases, data interpretations, mock exams, vivas and extensive course notes which provide:
* hundreds of high quality questions with detailed answers and explanations
* succinct notes, diagrams and charts

Personal attention:
Active participation is encouraged on these courses, so in order to give personal tuition and to answer individual questions our course numbers are limited. Book early to avoid disappointment.

Choice of courses:
PasTest has developed a wide range of high quality interactive courses in different cities around the UK to suit your individual needs.

What other candidates have said about our courses:
'Absolutely brilliant – I would not have passed without it! Thank you.'
Dr Charitha Rajapakse, London.

'Excellent, enjoyable, extremely hard work but worth every penny.'
Dr Helen Binns, Oxford.

For further details contact:
PasTest Ltd, Egerton Court, Parkgate Estate
Knutsford, Cheshire WA16 8DX, UK.
Telephone: 01565 752000 Fax: 01565 650264
e-mail: courses@pastest.co.uk web site: www.pastest.co.uk